An Illustrated Guide To Practical Sexual Positions

Everything You Need To Know For Wild Monkey Sex

by C.W. Pollard

Overunity Publications

Legal Disclaimer

Introduction

When you first start having sex, you are just happy to be doing it and you give little thought to all the possibilities that exist as to how men and women pair together. That doesn't last long. Once you have begun having sex, there is a strong desire to explore and see just how many ways you can find that we can fit together with no pieces left over.

This book was written to aid you in that quest. Now, there is nothing new about a sexual positions manual. The famous Indian love manuals were written thousands of years ago and stand as proof to humankind's enduring desire for knowledge on the subject.

However, based on my own experience, many of the love manuals that exist are full of impractical positions that you need to be a contortionist to appreciate. I'm not and I am willing to bet you aren't either. Chances are you are a horny man or woman that is set on seeing what practical possibilities exist for you in the bedroom.

Hopefully, this is what you are getting in this book. This is a book full of **practical** sexual positions. These positions are comfortable and can be assumed by anyone. You don't need any sex swings, straps, pulleys or cranes to make them work. Two horny people and a comfortable place will suffice.

In addition to not needing anything special to assume these positions, this book also will present in practical terms, the strengths and weaknesses of the positions in no nonsense, easy to understand terms.

This is exactly the book you need to spice up your bedroom antics and create a richer, more fulfilling, wilder and interesting sex life!

A Discussion Of The Difficulty Rating System Used

All of the positions in this book are achievable. Nothing here will push the human body beyond it's limits. However, all the positions are rated from easy to moderate to hard and I want to quickly define what those mean, in the context of this work.

Easy – An easy sexual position will require no work from the couple to maintain it. Once it is entered into nobody will have to work to keep their balance. There is no chance of falling over and the position is perfectly comfortable to everyone involved. These positions would be described as very natural sexual coupling positions.

Moderate – A moderately difficult sexual position involves more than this. It is going to take a little work from the couple. At least one member of the couple is going to need to work to maintain their balance. There is a chance of falling over onto the bed in the heat of passion. These are the positions you need to work a little bit at and may push parts of the body in ways it was not meant to bend, although not uncomfortably so.

Difficult – Difficult sexual positions, as far as this book is concerned are the positions that the couple needs to work together to maintain. They must work as a couple and coordinate their efforts. He must support her while she assumes a body form that is hard to keep going, or vice versa. There are not many of these positions in this book. However, these ones can be especially fun and the teamwork needed to make them happen only brings a couple closer together.

A Discussion Of The Intimacy Rating System Used

Intimacy is something that is hard to define, however, in discussing these positions, I had to include some indication as to how intimate they are. I have done so with a standard low, medium and high rating. Now this is largely based on my personal opinions, however you will find that positions with the same rating will share many common features.

Low – Positions that are described as low will usually not be face to face positions. Usually one partner is acting in a manner that is dominating to the other. Low intimacy positions also tend to be fast paced with lots of hard fucking.

Medium – Positions that have a medium intimacy level are usually face to face, but in a manner that is not permitting to kissing. The face to face adds to the intimacy, but the lack of kissing still keeps it low. Kissing after all is one of the key elements to highly intimate sex. These positions are also slower in pace, but tend to be more vigorous none the less.

High – Positions that are high in the intimacy rating tend to face to face in a way that the couple can make out a lot. The sexual positions that receive this rating are also usually high in body contact. The two of you will touch over a lot of your skin. Lastly, these positions are slow paced, with deep penetration that allows for slow, tender, soft lovemaking.

A Discussion Of The Wildness Rating System Used

Again, rating how "wild" a sexual position is is another big subjective. What is wild to one person is not wild to another. However, there is a pattern that will make this explanation brief.

Usually when a sexual position is low in intimacy, like a spontaneous blowjob in the women's room at a club, it is very wild. When a position is high in intimacy, it is usually not a hard fucking, back clawing, can't believe how strong that orgasm was kind of affair.

What this means is that intimacy and wildness are usually opposite. When one is high, the other is low, etc., etc.

I followed this pattern throughout this book. Now, you may not agree with me and you may think that some are wilder than I have indicated and others not so much. Again, this is subjective and is based on my perceptions. They were my calls and I have made them. However, you should always remember, that the only way to know for yourself what you think of these positions is to try them all out for yourself. Now, that is a bit of homework that I can get behind.

A Few Word On Female Orgasm For The Couple

In this book, each sexual position lists whether or not it is good for female orgasm. I want to write a few words discussing this.

First, of all I want to make sure that you, the reader, understands that I am only referring to clitoral orgasms. This is the type of orgasm that any woman can have, provided that her clit is stimulated correctly and she is relaxed enough.

Vaginal orgasms and the G-spot fall into the realm of the Sasquatch. They may very well be real, I will not argue that point. However, medical science has yet to demonstrate conclusively whether or not they are. Since this is the case, I am not going to focus on them. The clitoris is real, very easy to find, and very easy to use to make a woman orgasm. Just about 100% of sexually active women will have masturbated via their clit and I am sure that they will agree with me.

Now, all of the pussy eating positions in this book can be used to give a woman an orgasm. It simply requires stimulating her clit with your mouth. This is sometimes trickier than others, and those positions discuss that in detail. However, if you want to make a woman orgasm, this is your first place to start.

For those of you looking to learn more about pussy eating, please consult my other work <u>The Secret Art Of Eating Pussy : Tips & Tricks To Please Her Every Time</u> (ISBN 978-1463655631) available via all online retailers.

For the intercourse positions that list that they are good for female orgasm, you really have two choices and I am going to tell you about both. Both of these options involves direct clitoral stimulation during intercourse.

The easiest and most basic way to stimulate the clitoris (I'm going to assume you know where it is) is manually with fingers. This can be done either by her or by her lover and it is up to the couple to decide which is best given the position.

Either way, you should stimulate her clitoris using your index and middle fingers, as shown in the picture below.

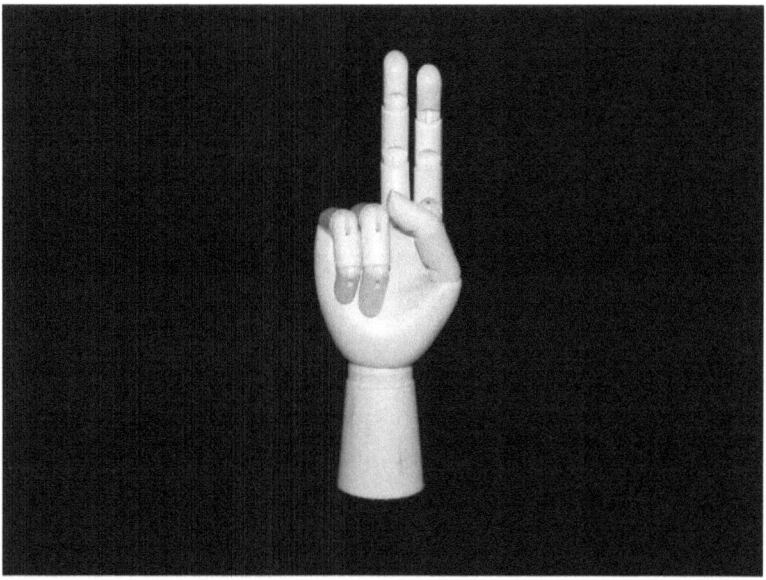

Men, if you are doing the fingering, make sure to lick your finger before you touch her pussy. I mean really lick it. Get it nice and wet with saliva, this will make sure everything is nice and lubricated and there won't be any chaffing of her delicate tissues.

Find her clit, and position your fingers so her clit is sitting right between your two fingers. Keep them together. Now, apply gentle pressure to her clit. Start light!!! You can always increase pressure as things heat up.

Start by rubbing her clit (this is all while you are inside her) in small circular motions. Like I said, start gentle and go from there. You can always get rougher and go faster. Start slow and gentle and pay attention to her reactions.

While you are doing this, apply gentle pressure into her vagina with your cock. You don't even have to really fuck her at this point. It is more than enough that you are inside her. Just move it in and out a little bit while you are doing what I said with your fingers. With a little luck she will be cumming in no time. Just pay attention to her!

Now some of the sexual positions that I describe may be a little tight and you may not have the full range of motion you need to give her an orgasm with your fingers. There are also other issues like the man being too aggressive and actually hurting her clit or his hand can cramp up. All of these are a problem.

Well, modern technology has come up with a solution that you cannot afford to ignore. Meet the "bullet" style vibrator. These very small vibrators address all of these problems. They are small enough to get in the tightest squeezes (no pun intended) and they never cramp up. They will provide constant, uninterrupted consistent stimulation to her clit while intercourse is going on. They are a tool that should be in the nightstand table for any sexually satisfied couple, or even single.

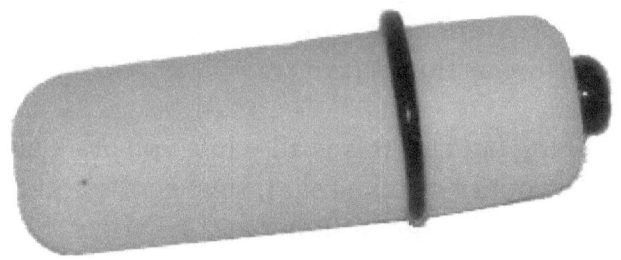

Shown <u>larger</u> than actual size.

Now, I have to mention that you, the man, can finger her or stimulate her with a vibrator. However, we live in enlightened times and I want you to know that she can do it too. There is absolutely nothing wrong with her fingering her clit or using a vibrator on her while the two of you are having sex. In fact, you should look at it as a good thing. For one, she is open enough to do that in front of you. Two, it is really sexy to watch. Three, it will make her cum and that is really the goal here. Lastly, sex will be more fulfilling, wilder when it happens and will happen more often.

Remember, the goal is a rosy cheeked, sexually satisfied woman. Nothing more, but certainly nothing less. You just want it to happen. How it happens is really just a minor detail. That's my advice. Take it or leave it.

<u>Anal And Lesbians....Oh My!</u>

I want to take a minute here to discuss anal sex and lesbians.

I would like to point out that with very few exceptions, all of the intercourse positions listed in this book can be easily adapted to anal sex. This applies to heterosexual and homosexual couples alike.

Additionally, for any lesbian couples that may purchase this work, all of the intercourse positions will work as well for you as heterosexual or gay couples. You will simply need to add a strap on dildo into the equation. However, with this minor addition, you will be able to enjoy the full range of positions that are listed in this book..

Additionally, for lesbian couples, you will find two positions that are specifically intended for you. Enjoy!

Is This An Exhaustive List Of Sexual Positions?

No! This work is by no means an exhaustive list of sexual positions. The human body is capable of contorting and fucking in many, many different ways.

This work, however, is designed to be a **practical** lesson in sexual positions. The positions that you will find in this book are intended to be the basic "moves" that you should be familiar with. Start with these. Get good at them and there is no telling how far you can go!

Part 1
Oral Sex Positions

The Assmuncher

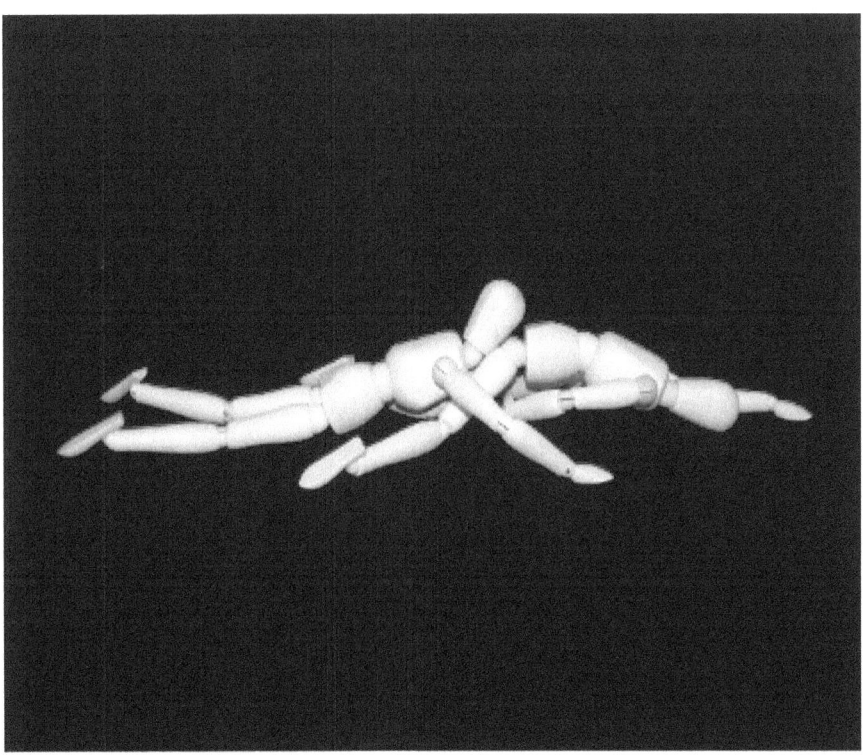

Position Description:

To assume the Assmuncher position, the woman lies on her stomach with her legs fully extended. Next she spreads her legs so that her feet are as wide apart as her shoulders. Now she arches her back. This has the effect of revealing her pussy and ass to her lover. He or she can now lick, suck and tickle her in any number of ways.

Ease Of Position: Easy

Intimacy Level: Moderate

Wild Spontaneous Level: Moderate

Depth Of Penetration: Not Applicable

Good For Female Orgasm? Yes

Upsides:

This position is a lot of fun. There is a lot of stimulation for her as well as attention. This is definitely one that is versatile. You can use this position as part of foreplay to get her wet. You can also go into this position straight from doggystyle by her extending her legs, or into it doggy from it by retracting them.

There is also a lot of visual stimulation for him. He gets up close with her pussy and optionally, her ass. There is lots of playing around and this is a definite turn on to most men and women.

Downsides:

The only real downside to this sexual position is the ass. What I mean by this is for her, her ass is out there on display and a lot of women are a bit bashful about their brown eyes. Also, when a man is licking her pussy in this position, his nose is right up close and personal with her ass. In both cases, this position may stretch the comfort level for one or both partners.

Notes On This Position:

This position is a great one to use during foreplay. All of the attention is focused on stimulating the woman. Her partner has full, unfettered access to both her pussy and ass. This allows for lots of possibilities in terms of licking, sucking and fingering.

As far as female orgasm in concerned, this is not a good position to orally stimulate her clitoris, and thus, oral sex to orgasm is difficult. The fact is that in this position, her clit is at a bit of a tricky angle for mouth stimulation. However, her clitoris is at a good angle for her to stimulate it either manually, or with a vibrator as discussed in the introduction.

On The Knees Blowjob

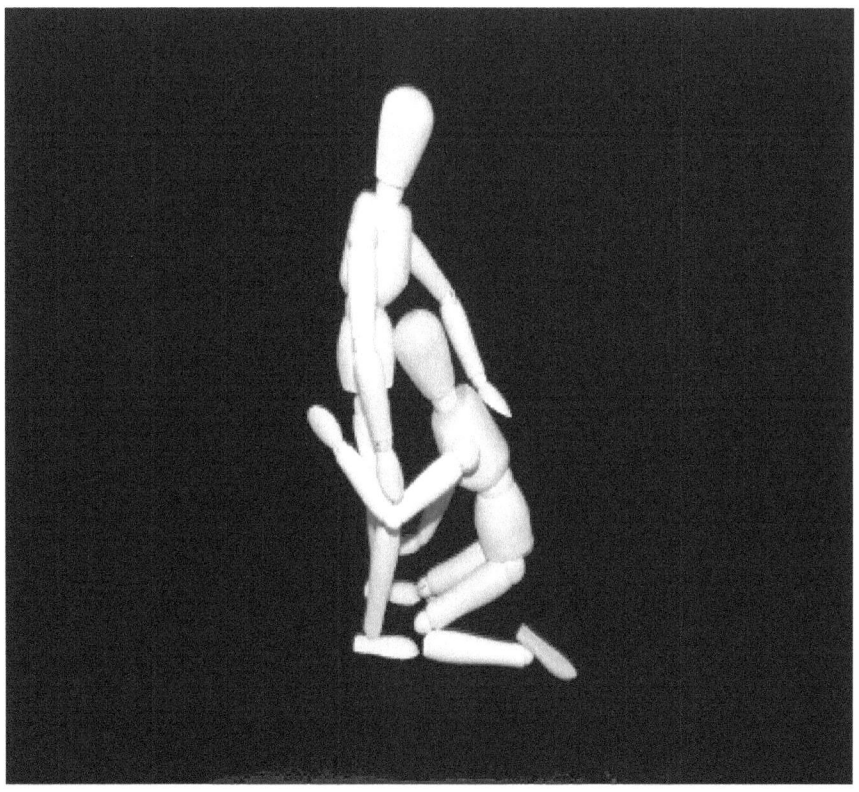

Position Description:

When people think of "blowjob" this is often what they have in mind. The woman gets on her knees in front of the man, facing him. At this level, she is eye to eye with his cock and balls. She can then engage in any and all types of fellatio she deems appropriate.

Ease Of Position: Moderate

Intimacy Level: Low

Wild Spontaneous Level: High

Good For Female Orgasm? No

Downsides:

One of the downsides to this position is a potential lack of intimacy. Notice that I said "potential". A woman performing this act can feel a little distant from her lover. There is the potential for her to feel cheap as well. However, to some this is the appeal of the act. The man definitely appears to dominate her in this act. A good way to combat this and for the couple to feel connected is to maintain eye contact. Eye contact communicates much even though she is not able to speak.

This position is also difficult for many men to orgasm in. He has to maintain his balance which may be difficult when he is cumming or may even interfere with him getting there. Lean against something if you can.

Upsides:

For him, he feels dominant. She is on her knees pleasuring him. This makes him feel powerful and in charge. For her, the reality is that she may be on her knees, but she does have his balls in her hands. Whatever the appearance, she is truly in control of this act and his pleasure.

This position also offers a great deal through its spontaneous nature. It can be performed for just a minute or two, even while out on the town, as part of a long term foreplay and teasing. This is her ultimate position for teasing when she wants to keep his attention on her or give him a raging case of blue balls.

Notes On This Position:

This is a very common and easy blowjob position. It can be very spontaneous. It works equally well when a couple ducks into an alley or a public bathroom stall as it does in the bedroom. It can be performed both clothed or nude. It also offers options in terms of the blow job itself. The couple can engage in mouth fucking, or she can be in total control.

<u>Standard Pussy Eating Position</u>

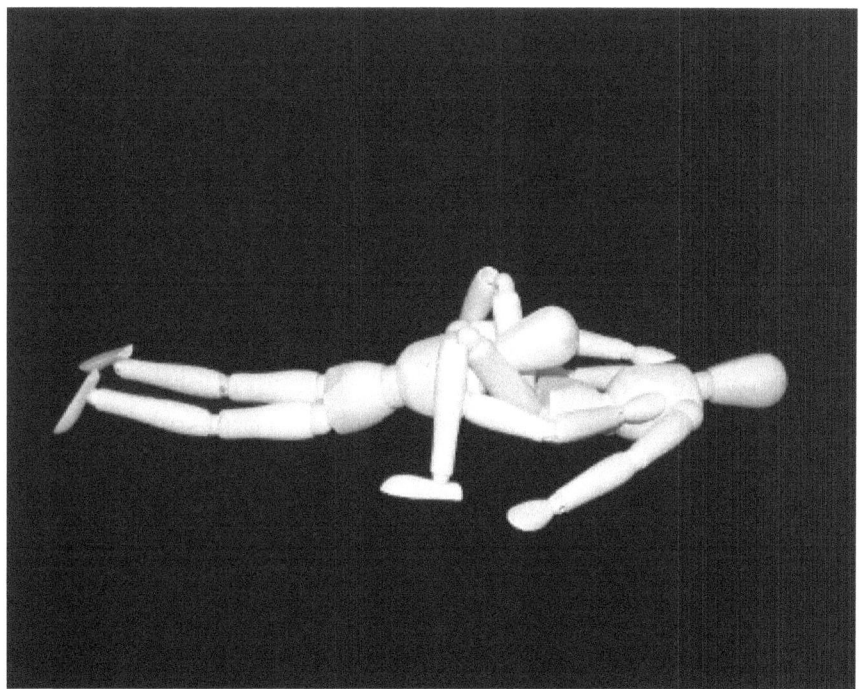

Position Description:

In this position the woman lies on her back on something comfortable. This is usually a bed although I have made it work on a sectional couch too.. She spreads her legs revealing her pussy to him. He then lies down with his face between her legs. He is in the perfect position to finger her while at the same time stimulating her clitoris with his mouth.

Ease Of Position: Easy

Intimacy Level: High

Wild Spontaneous Level: Moderate

Good For Female Orgasm? Yes

Notes On This Position:

For cunnilingus, this position is it! She is lying down and able to relax, while her lover has total access to all of her sensitive bits. This being said, he can pleasure her to orgasm easily. With her legs bent and her feet flush on the surface of the bed, she is able to move her hips and pelvis to help bring her clit and vagina into the right position to meet and aid his stimulation.

This position is also very intimate. She is in a position to look down on her lover and see him pleasuring her and focusing all his attention on her. He can look up and meet her eyes. Maintaining eye contact will increase this.

Upsides:

The upside to this position is her comfort and mobility. She can relax and receive the pleasure easily. She is also able to move her hips to bring her clit to the maximum level of stimulation.

Also, her ass is discretely tucked back and is out of the way. This is a plus to those women who are a little sensitive about their asses being out on display.

Downsides:

This position really doesn't have any downsides. It is the perfect position for pussy eating and should be used to make her cum often!

Undercarriage Work

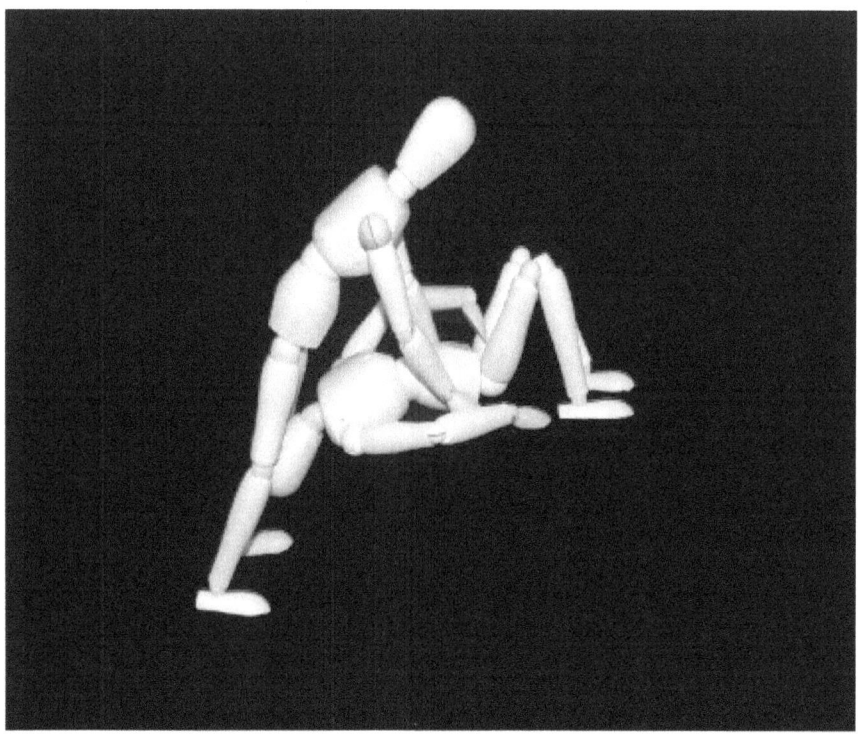

Position Description:

This is a fellatio sexual position. In this position, the woman lies on a bed face up with her head hanging off. The man then comes close as though to straddle her face. He lets her be in control, he just stands there and allows her to pleasure him. If she decides to, she can take his whole cock into her mouth. Her throat is in the perfect position for deep throating.

If this is the case, she can guide him in and control his hip movement by placing her hands on his butt cheeks. In this way, he can fuck her mouth until orgasm or until they switch positions.

There is also the option, since her clitoris is easily accessible for self stimulation or toy stimulation. The man can also easily play with and stimulate her clitoris, although finger penetration can be hard to achieve.

If clit stimulation is decided on, make it non-goal oriented foreplay. The goal of an orgasm will only complicate things too much.

Ease Of Position: Moderate

Intimacy Level: Low

Wild Spontaneous Level: High

Good For Female Orgasm? Impractical

Downsides:

There is a possibility of the man getting to excited and beginning to penetrate her mouth to a depth and at a speed that is uncomfortable to her. This can result in gagging and discomfort. To avoid this, if his cock is in her mouth, she should have at least one hand on the shaft to control depth until the couple finds a good rhythm.

Upsides:

This position is very visually and physically stimulating for the man. He will be talking about it for days!

Notes On This Position:

There is an element of domination and control at play with this position. He may feel dominant and this is a turn on to him. However, like the kneeling blowjob, she again is in total control (even though he may not realize it). Couples who enjoy an element of dominance and submission will really enjoy this one. Also, women who enjoy the act of fellatio will find this act to be a novel twist on an old favorite.

This position is also versatile in that it can be foreplay to actual sex, or it can be the main sex act, or a follow up after intercourse.

Dominant Blowjob

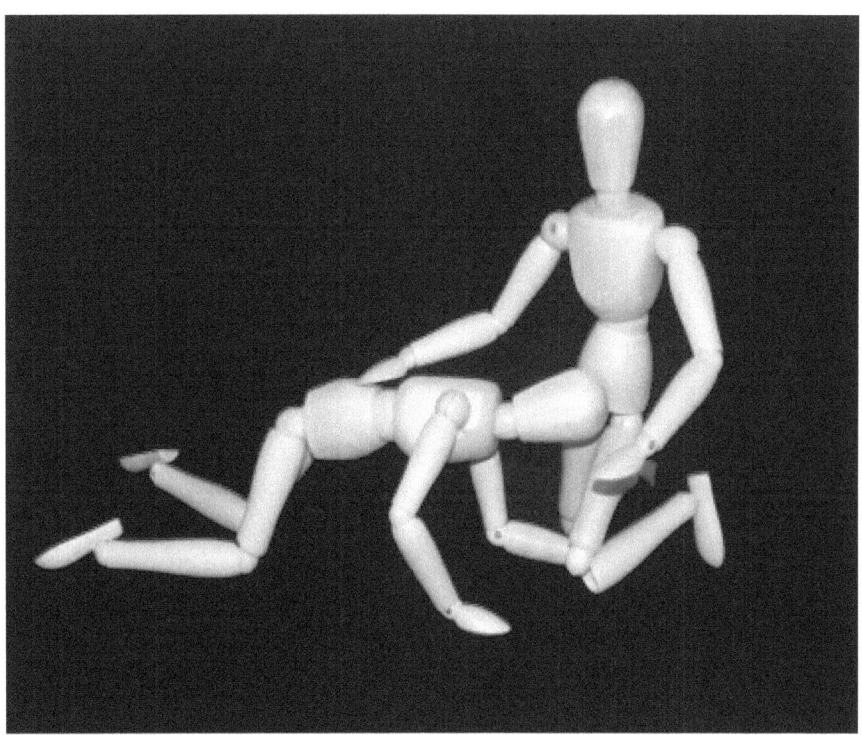

Position Description:

In the dominant blowjob position, the woman is on all fours and the man is on his knees towering over her. He can be directly in front of her, or to the side. His cock is right in her face. She can easily engage in a blowjob at this point. If she chooses to, she can shift her weight to just one hand and manually stroke his cock as well.

He, on the other hand, can lean over her and play with her breasts, spank her, engage in ass play, or even finger her if his arms are long enough.

Ease Of Position: Moderate

Intimacy Level: Low

Wild Spontaneous Level: High

Good For Female Orgasm? No

Downsides:

This position puts high demands on the woman's neck. If she remains in this position too long, she can suffer discomfort and stiffness later. The other downside, as is common with mouthfucking, is that the man can get a little to into the action and begin thrusting. If he becomes over enthusiastic, he can go too deep and cause discomfort and gagging.

Upsides:

This position has the man in the dominant position while his woman is giving him pleasure. As such, this can be a positive to both partners in the dominance category. She will feel very much that he is in control. Also, because of the position, he is able to stimulate her a bit. This involves him in the action and helps to make this position a fun one for foreplay.

Notes On This Position:

I am going to be honest. This position is really one that was dreamed up by a man. He is in control and dominant. She is on her knees. He has access to her breasts, pussy and ass. He can mouthfuck her. Lastly, it is a visual feast for him. He gets to look down on her with his cock in her mouth and see all of her sexy curves. The passion and desire will overcome him quickly. This position does tend to shift quickly to actual intercourse.

This is not to say that she can't have a ball with his cock in her mouth, but he is almost certain to smiling after the two of you perform this little number.

As with all mouthfucking positions, if the woman can, she should put a hand around the shaft of his cock. This will act like a check in the event he gets to enthusiastic and will prevent him from thrusting too deep.

Basic Orgasm Blowjob

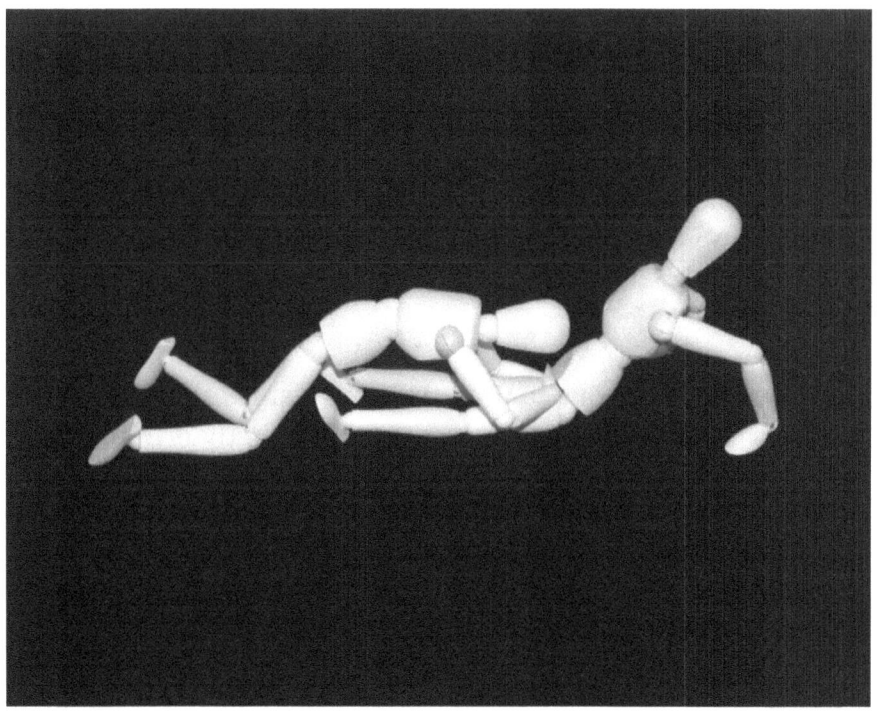

Position Description:

In this position the man lies down on the bed. The woman, in the doggystyle position, crawls over him so his cock is even with her mouth. She then is in position to perform a thorough blowjob.

Ease Of Position: Easy

Intimacy Level: High

Wild Spontaneous Level: Moderate

Good For Female Orgasm? No

Downsides:

If this blowjob goes on for a long time her arms can go a bit numb. This is the only appreciable downside to this position.

Upsides:

This position is the one to use when she wants to give him a long, pleasurable blowjob to orgasm. Everybody is in the right position. Everyone is pretty comfortable. She is able to support herself with one arm easily to add manual stimulation to the blowjob she is performing with her mouth.

Notes On This Position:

This is called the basic blowjob position because there are no frills, but it will get the job done every time. It is best performed in the comfort of bed, but will work most other places the two of you can sprawl out on as well.

He should get good and comfortable. This can mean he lies on his back, but it is really better is he is sitting up a bit, propped against a pillow. In the blowjob, there is a lot more going on than just a cock in her mouth and the pleasure from that. There is a ton of visual stimulation that one can miss out on unless they are sitting up and watching. He gets to see her mouth and head going up and down. There is her sexy hair. There is the even sexier eye contact that adds a playful, seductive, even coquettish note to the act. If he is sitting up, he can touch and caress.

One word for the guys – don't put your hand on the back of her head until she tells you to do it. Some women can find that a bit rude and it will cause a quick end to the blowjob.

For her, this act has several uses. She can use it as a part of foreplay. Nothing will get your man ready for sex faster than the soft touch of your mouth. On the other hand, you can use this as a finisher too.

Say you are in the cowgirl position that will be discussed later (you can skip ahead if you want to peek), well, you can slide down from that position and easily tease him orally for a minute. You can then go into another sexual position, or you can just as easily give him a teasingly slow blowjob to orgasm. Your call.

I did mark this position as not good for female orgasm. There is some truth to that, but you are welcome to give it a go. Most women will have trouble giving him a blowjob to orgasm while they are playing with their clit's to climax. On the other hand, there is nothing that says you cannot play with your clit to orgasm while you are giving him a slow, even lackadaisical blowjob. Finish him off when you're done if you think he's earned it. He can wait his turn for once.

The Coquettish Blowjob

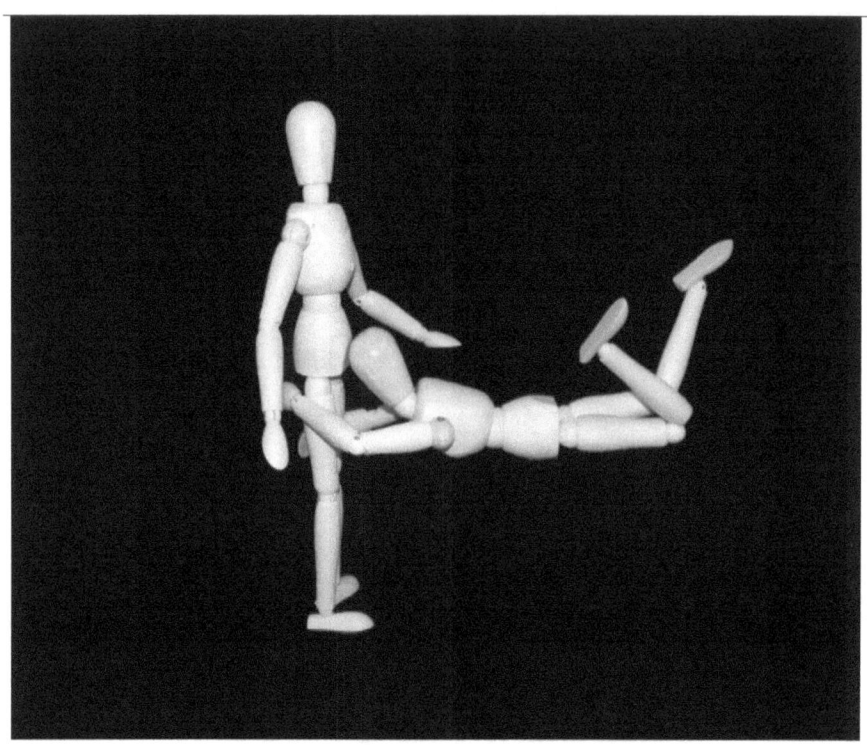

Position Description:

In this position, the woman lies on the bed face down. The man stands at the end of the bed and approaches her. She arches her back and raises her head to be on level with his cock. To help in doing this, she can rest he weight on her elbows. In this way, her hands are free to help her while performing fellatio.

Ease Of Position: Easy

Intimacy Level: Moderate To High

Wild Spontaneous Level: Low

Good For Female Orgasm? No

Downsides:

The only downside to this position is that her neck can become sore from strain after too long. If he does approach orgasm, his balance can become unsteady as well. If this occurs, he may land on her if he falls.

Upsides:

This is a very intimate oral sex position that can be very slow paced and tender. This position also offers him lots of visual stimulation while she is pleasuring him. He gets to stare down at her lovely ass, which is after all one of the greatest visual sex attractants.

Notes On This Position:

This is a very playful and coquettish position for a blowjob. She is reclined, stretched out and relaxed. He is standing over her, waiting to see what she will do next. The woman can use this to her advantage, as well as the pleasure of both. She can use the visual stimulation, combined with slow oral sex to tease him. His desires will be awakened and his lust will begin to bubble toward the boiling point. How long can he manage before he must have her?

This position is also a good one for mouthfucking. This can be vigorous, or it can be used as part of a slow, teasing bit of oral sex foreplay. With her hands free she is in a good position to grab his ass to set the pace of any thrusting, as well as to control the depth.

This position is usually best before actual intercourse. Once intercourse has commenced, the teasing that makes this position so much fun becomes a lot harder.

Lick Me!

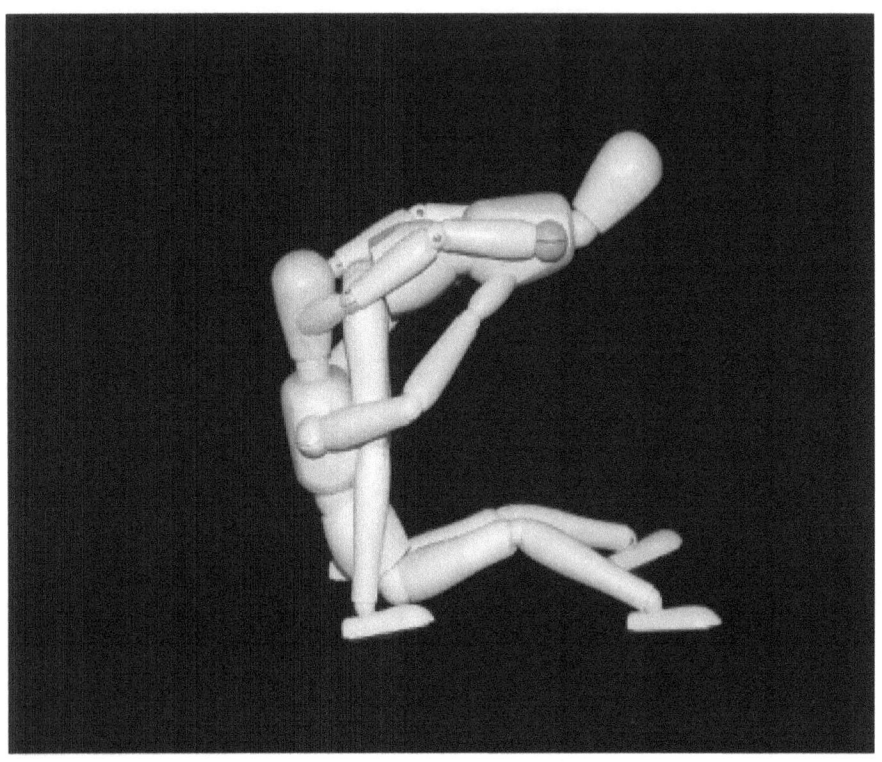

Position Description:

This is a pussy eating position. In this position, the woman stands in front of the man while he is seated on the floor. She spreads her legs about shoulder width apart. She then backs up and grabs his head. She pulls his face into her pussy and calls out "Lick Me!" He then does as he is told while she barks out commands.

Ease Of Position: Easy

Intimacy Level: Moderate

Wild Spontaneous Level: High

Good For Female Orgasm? Yes

Downsides:

In this position, like most standing positions, the woman's legs can grow tired. Also, as she moves towards orgasm, her balance may not hold and she can fall.

Upsides:

In this position, the man has full access to all of the woman's erogenous zones. He is in the position to offer significant oral stimulation. This position is also a pussy eating position that puts the woman in the dominant role. This can be a huge plus.

Notes On This Position:

Up to this point, most of the oral sex positions that have been discussed have put the man in the dominant position. This position (and the one that follows) offer the ladies a chance to exercise their dominance over their partners.

This can actually be a positive or a negative depending on the couple. In many cases, women enjoy taking a dominant role in the bedroom. Well in this position, she is playfully forcing her lover to pleasure her, complete with a hand on the back of his head for good measure.

If you are a woman reading this, you should give this position and the following at least a try. See if you like them. If you don't you are always welcome to drop them from your sexual routine. But you never know until you try.

As to her orgasm, this position certainly does put all the components together for a woman's orgasm. He is right there on her clit and she is guiding him. She will most likely need to move her hips to help him find the perfect angle for her. This position is also great as a non-orgasm, foreplay only position.

If the couple is going to seek orgasm, it would be best to perform this act in a place that allows her to lean on something for comfort. This will also help her relax and surrender to her building orgasm. Anything will work but most convenient in the bedroom would be a dresser, bed frame or wall.

Get To Work Sailor

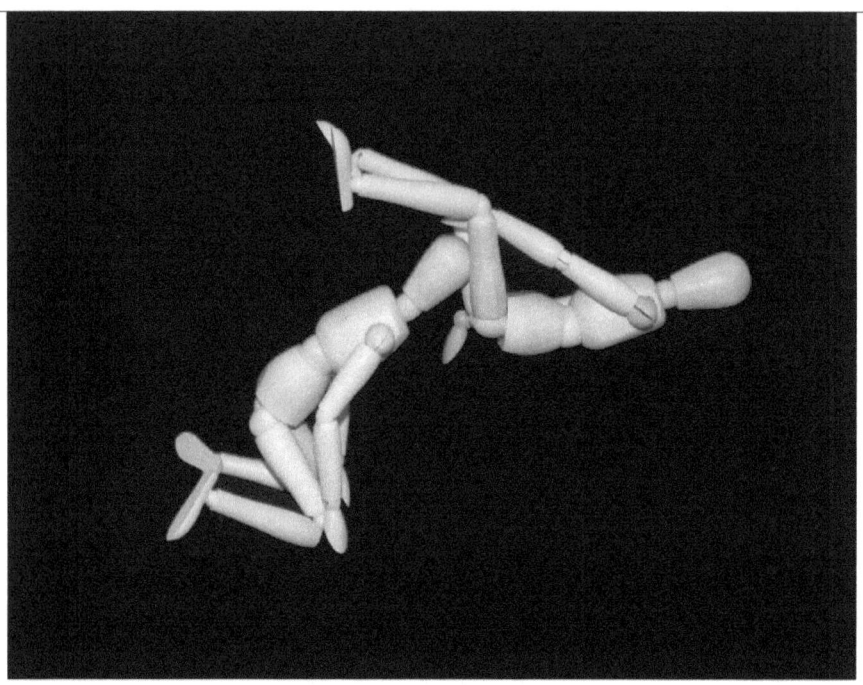

Position Description:

In this position, the woman sits on a surface that is between knee and waist high, with her legs dangling over the edge. Common furniture solutions to this problem include the bed, couch, and recliner. Now, it is important that the surface that she is reclining on be padded. She may be there for a while and the padding will help to keep her comfortable. Also, the fabric will help to soak up, and hide any wet spots that are created.

Once she has laid back she spreads he legs and bends them at the knee. It is important to be clear that her legs are not on the surface that she is lying on, but instead are in the air. The same is true for her feet.

Once she has assumed this position, her lover approaches her on his hands and knees and begins to give her oral sex.

Ease Of Position: Moderate

Intimacy Level: High

Wild Spontaneous Level: High

Good For Female Orgasm? Yes

Downsides:

With her legs in the air, she can grow tired fairly easily. The man can help with this by placing his hands on the underside of her thighs. This will give her extra support and allow her to relax, although it will make fingering during oral sex difficult.

Upsides:

This position exposes all of her her erogenous zones to the man's attentions. No bit of sensitive skin is beyond his pleasuring. Also, she is in control and is dominant again. She is lying back and letting him do all the work up to and including bearing the weight of her legs.

Notes On This Position:

This position is a great cunnilingus position. There is real ease of access and she is in a pretty comfortable position. What may not be apparent at first is that this position is an easy one to transition to or from intercourse. That makes for a nice continuity of sex.

For example, assume that you are engaged in missionary position sex on a bed. Well, it is very easy for the man to go right into this position and then transition right into a "Double Handed Buttlift" without skipping a beat. All he has to do is pull the woman a few inches one way and get to licking.

The Big Boss

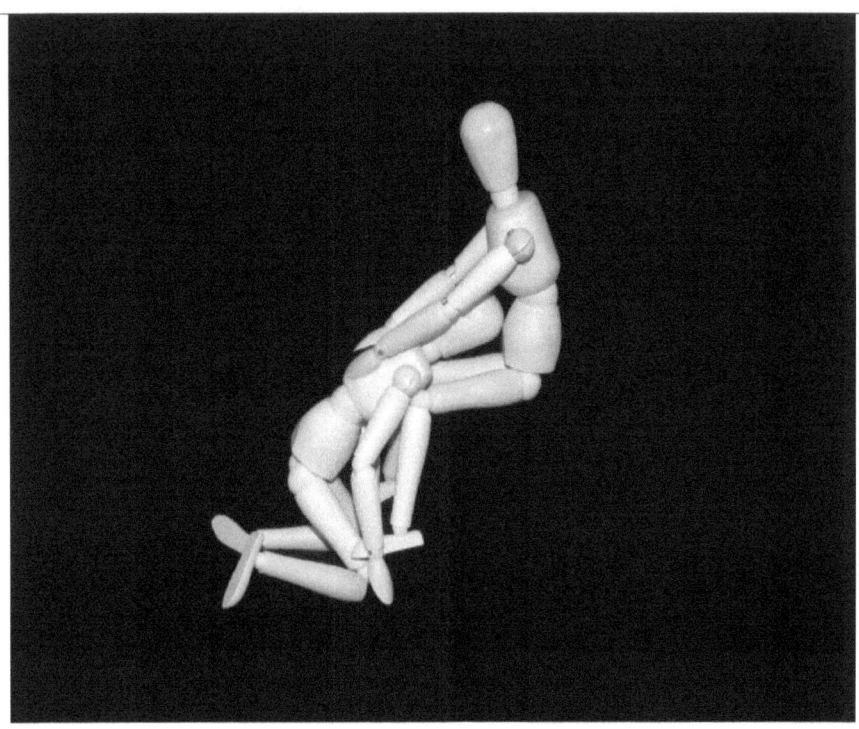

Position Description:

The "Big Boss" is a position that works equally well for pussy eating or a blowjob. In either permutation, the person who is going to receive oral sex sits in a chair. If the position is going to be used for pussy eating, it is easier if the chair does not have arms. This will allow the woman to spread her legs more fully. If the chair does have arms, she will most likely need to throw her legs over them. For some women, this may be uncomfortable.

Once the recipient is in seated, the oral sex giver gets on their knees and proceeds to pleasure their partner.

Ease Of Position: Easy

Intimacy Level: Moderate

Wild Spontaneous Level: High

Good For Female Orgasm? Yes

Downsides:

The only downside to this position is that if the chair has arms, the woman's legs need to be thrown over the arms. If the pussy eating goes on for a while, her legs can become uncomfortable.

Upsides:

This position is a very convenient oral sex position. It works equally well for cunnilingus and fellatio. It is also really easy to pull off spontaneously. It works very well with the furniture that is found in a typical office. This can easily lead to some naughty workplace fun for lovers. One partner can easily crawl under a desk and make the other smile.

If the couple plans on this ahead of time, it makes things much easier if the woman has a skirt on.

Notes On This Position:

The Big boss is a fun oral sex position for men and women. There is a lot of fun in either part of this. Looking up subserviently at the person in the chair is a thrill. Being on your knees while they moan with pleasure is always a turn on.

This is another one of those positions that you need to remember when you and your partner start messing around in the living room with all those plush chairs!

Aristocratic Pussy Eating

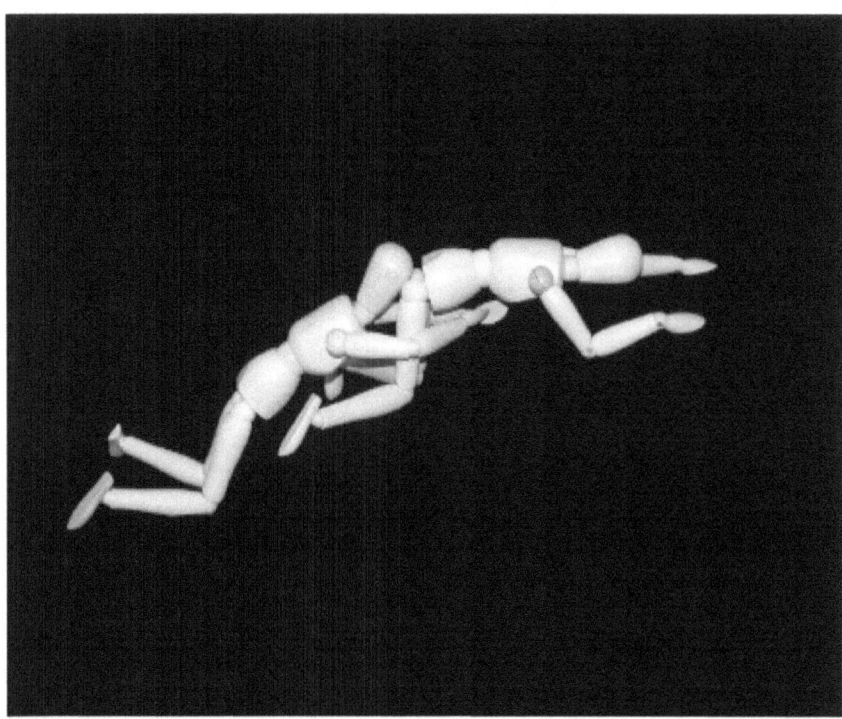

Position Description:

This position requires a piece of furniture like a couch or a recliner. Sectionals are just wonderful for an afternoon of wild monkey, sex play and work perfectly for this position.

Once the piece of furniture has been identified the woman climbs onto it and assumes the doggystyle position. Removing her clothing is optional in this position. She is welcome to either drop her pants or lift her skirt to allow access to her vulva.

The man then approaches her from behind on his knees. He should be on the floor, not the furniture. From here he can lick both her pussy and ass to her delight.

Ease Of Position: Easy

Intimacy Level: Moderate

Wild Spontaneous Level: High

Depth Of Penetration: N/A

Good For Female Orgasm? Yes

Downsides:

There are no appreciable downsides to this position. It is fun for all!

Upsides:

This position is a lot of fun. There is definitely a spirit of play and fun that everyone should experience.

There is also a sense that the man is simply there to pleasure the woman while she relaxes and enjoys. She is just there letting him do his work. This is empowering and hedonistic for her.

The spontaneity of this position is a big plus too. As long as you have a high enough surface you can do it anywhere, quickly. This makes it the ideal position to assume just before company comes over. It can be your dirty little secret the rest of the party.

Notes On This Position:

This position is a great one for a mid-afternoon sexual interlude. The two of you have been ignoring the river of passion that flows between you until the dam breaks. She lifts her skirt, assumes the position and tells him to get to work. He does with joy in his heart.

This is also a great transitional position. After she has hiked her skirt and he has eaten her pussy through several orgasms, he can stand up, drop his pants to his ankles and quickly insert himself into her for some vigorous fucking. This can take a while or the whole thing can be over in 20 minutes making it an ideal "quickie position".

The Spirit Of '69

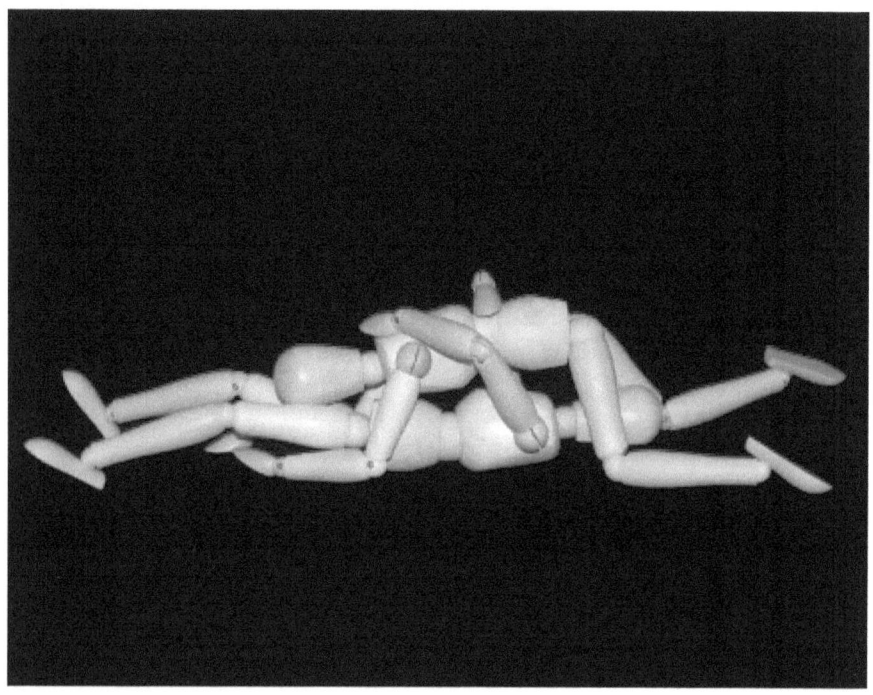

Position Description:

This position has two incarnations. Either partner can be on top.

With the woman on top, the man lies on the bed with his feet stretched out. She the straddles his face and leans down to engage in fellatio. He in turn lifts his head to begin orally stimulating her pussy.

The position with the man on top is similar, yet subtly different. She lies on the bed, however, instead of outstretching her legs (this would make her pussy inaccessible), she places the soles of her feet together. This spreads her legs in a comfortable position. He then straddles her face and leans forward to begin stimulating her pussy. She in turn begin to orally stimulate his cock and balls.

Ease Of Position: Easy

Intimacy Level: High

Wild Spontaneous Level: High

Depth Of Penetration: N/A

Good For Female Orgasm? Possible, but can be difficult

Downsides:

The only appreciable downside to this position is that the person on the bottom usually has their nose right in their partner's ass. For some this is a turn off. For others, this is a turn on.

Upsides:

This position is high in stimulation. It is fun to give oral sex. It is fun to get oral sex. This position actually adds the two together. If one is good two can be even better.

Notes On This Position:

Few sexual positions elicit the attention of the '69. It is really a subject unto itself in popular culture. That being said, almost every couple should give it a try at least once. It can really be a lot of fun for everyone involved. There is lots of oral stimulation which is physically pleasing. There is also a lot of giving oral sex which is emotionally pleasing as well. Lastly, there is also a lot of visual stimulation which is appreciated by both sexes.

One point that I want to make is that this position is not the easiest as far as female orgasm goes. First off, in this position, she is never in a very good position for you to orally stimulate her clitoris. You can stimulate it, but you will often have to strain. There is also the the problem of attention. She is getting her pussy licked, and he is usually getting his dick sucked. Neither partner is in a really good position to either focus on what they are doing or relax and enjoy what is being done to them enough to orgasm. Generally, this position is best for mutual oral sex as a foreplay act only. If either partner wants to make the other cum, refer to the other oral sex positions that are suggested in this book.

If, on the other hand, the couple is dead set on making her cum in this position (he should be able too with little coaxing), try the position with her on top (performing fellatio) and him on bottom using a small vibrator on her clitoris. Focused or not, a vibrator is usually enough to make her cum quickly.

Mouthfucking

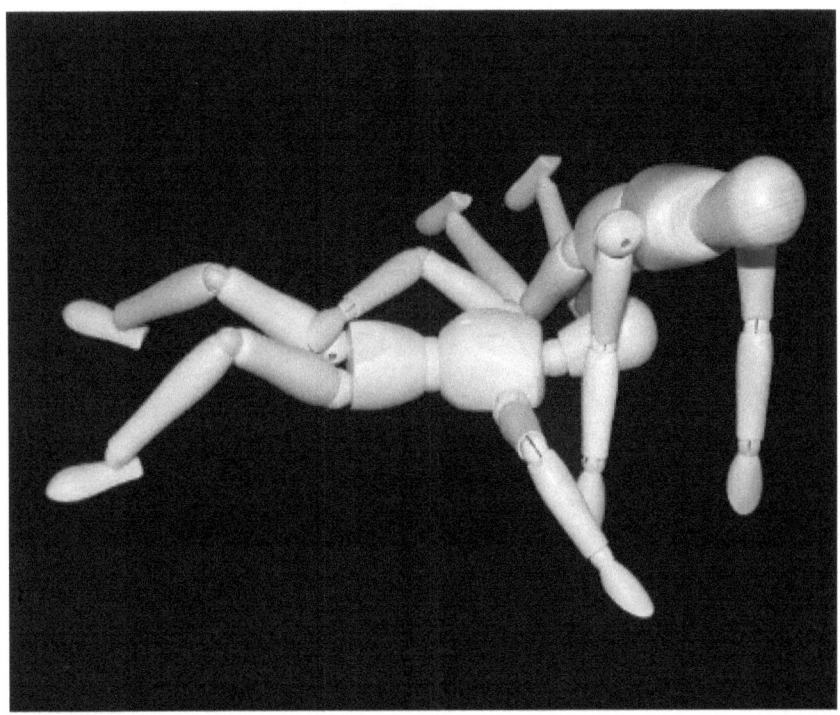

Position Description:

In this position the woman lies on the bed. The man then assumes a four point position over her face.

She should take hold of his cock at this point and place it in her mouth. He is now in a position to literally fuck her mouth and can do so by simply moving his hips in and out.

Ease Of Position: Easy

Intimacy Level: Low

Wild Spontaneous Level: High

Depth Of Penetration: N/A

Good For Female Orgasm? Yes

Downsides:

It is very easy for any man to get carried away and get too rough. Although a mouth can be fucked, they are not specifically designed for that. This means if he goes to deep he can easily cause her to gag. To avoid this problem, it is not a bad idea for the woman to keep a hand on his cock. This will create a block that will prevent him from going to deep.

Upsides:

Lots of women really enjoy the dominant aspect of this position. In fact, since the man is doing the majority of the work, the woman is very free to play with her clit with either a vibrator of her fingers. This will only increase the visual stimulation for the man. The two of you can enjoy some very strong orgasms from this combination of factors.

Notes On This Position:

If you are going to engage in this position, it is best that the woman be comfortable with the man cumming in her mouth. Trying to pull out or stop when he is close is probably going to be too much for him the first time you try this very sexy position. Just putting that out there.

Other than that, this is a fun position that should definitely be tried by more sexually adventurous couples.

Face Sitting

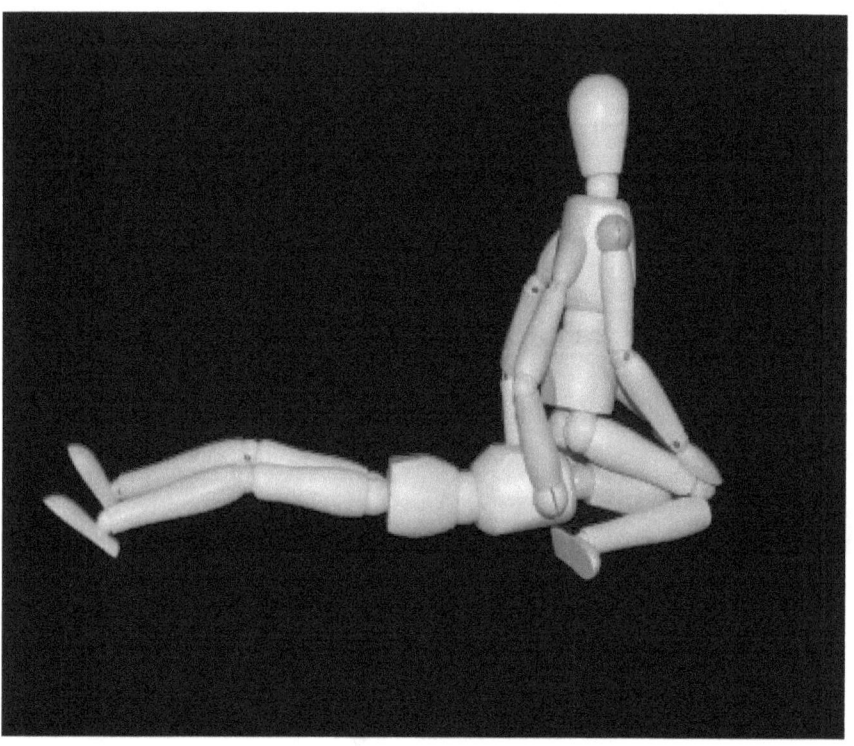

Position Description:

In this position, the man lies on the bed or floor and the woman straddles his face. She rests her weight on her knees and feet. The man's arms should be all the way behind the woman. In this way, he can support her as she leans back (if desired).

Ease Of Position: Easy

Intimacy Level: Moderate

Wild Spontaneous Level: Moderate

Depth Of Penetration: N/A

Good For Female Orgasm? Yes

Downsides:

The only appreciable downside to this position is that the woman's legs can get sore after a while.

Upsides:

There is a lot of visual stimulation for the man. This can be a huge turn on.

Notes On This Position:

This position puts the woman on top of the man's mouth. However, her legs are cocked back. This gives her a tremendous amount of control over her hips. With this control, she can easily move her clit however she needs to so he is constantly stimulating it. She is also in the right position to bear down or lift up her clit. This means not only is she in control over how her clit is being stimulated, she is also in control of the pressure on it.

For women whose partners have trouble finding her clit during oral sex, or perhaps are too rough when they do, this position is a wonderful tool. It takes the guesswork out of their hands and will get her off.

For the man, he needs to focus less on moving and more on maintaining a continuous and steady form of stimulation. Don't move after her clit, but instead trust her movement and let her bring her clit to you.

One potential issue with this position is that the woman needs to maintain balance. This can be made much easier by positioning her at the head of a bed. Usually she will find either a headboard or a wall that she can lean on. This, in combination with her lovers supporting hands, should make her plenty steady and allow her to relax enough to really get into the pussy eating.

There is also the option for her to go down on all fours. This will not make her clit inaccessible and will also make her good and steady.

The Sneak Attack

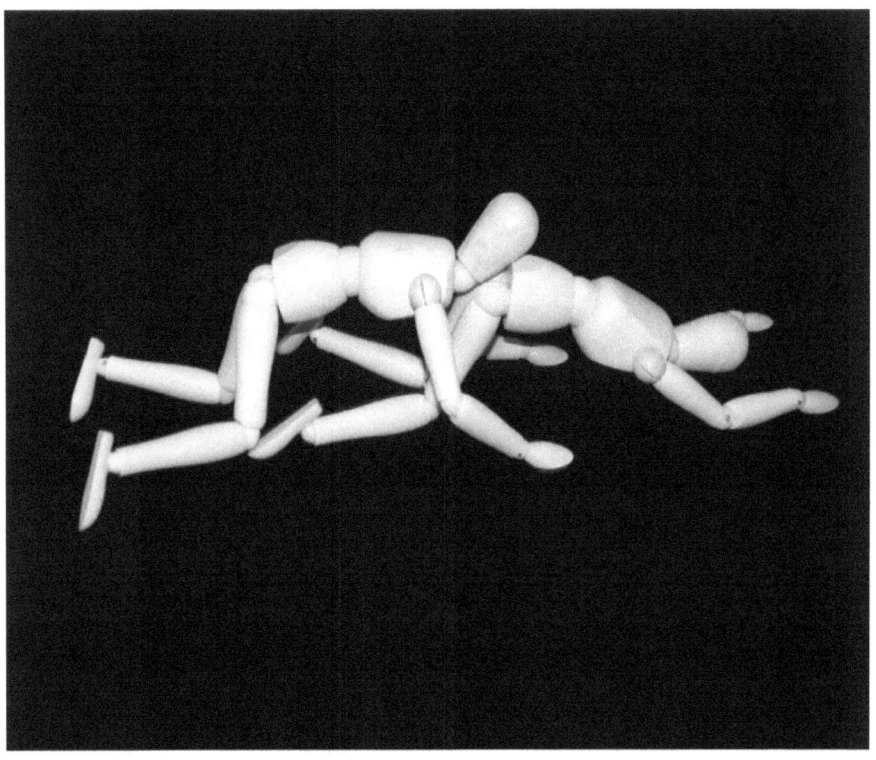

Position Description:

With the sneak attack, both partners are in the doggystyle position. The woman is in front. The man comes up behind her. Both her pussy and ass are exposed. He is now able to orally stimulate all of her hotspots without having to move.

Ease Of Position: Easy

Intimacy Level: High

Wild Spontaneous Level: High

Depth Of Penetration: N/A

Good For Female Orgasm? Yes and No

Downsides:

The downside of this position is that his nose is very close to her exposed ass. This can be a sticky point for him if he is inexperienced with assplay, or is squeamish. This can also be a problem if she is uncomfortable with assplay as he is most likely going to be tempted to pleasure her there in some way.

Upsides:

This oral sex position offers easy access to all the tantalizing treasures that are found between a woman's legs. The man is also somewhat submissive to her. He is on his knees just licking away for her pleasure. This can be a real turn on for both partners.

Notes On This Position:

Orgasm with this position is a bit tricky. Since the man approaches the clitoris from above, he is not in the best position to offer consistent stimulation. This can make it hard for him to make her cum. Now, on the other hand, this can be an ideal position for her to play with her clit until she cums while he licks her pussy and ass. That can be a lot of fun.

This position can also be a transitional, quick position. The couple can easily engage in this position before or after doggystyle while they are switching to another position. The couple can also easily go from doggystyle to the sneak attack and then back to doggystyle without her having to move at all. This offers her a wide variety of stimulation that can't fail to make and keep her hot! It is up to both of you to figure out how this works into your sexual routine.

Part 2
Intercourse Sexual Positions

Bent Over With One Leg Up

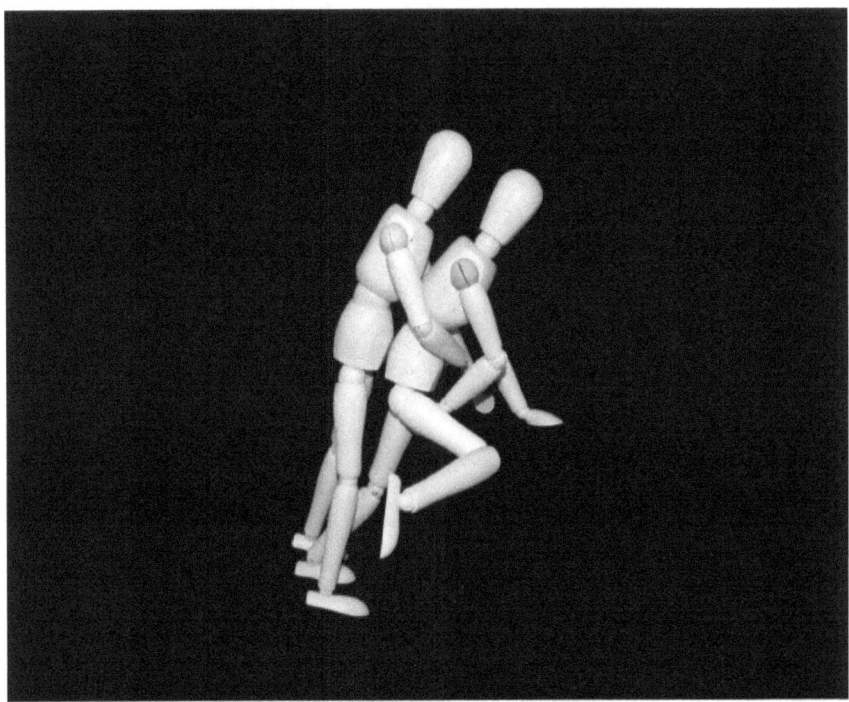

Position Description:

This is a variation on the "Bend Her Over Something" position.

The couple begins just like in that position, however, the woman lifts one of her legs and rests it on whatever she is being bent over. This has the effect of opening her legs and supporting her at the same time. In doing so she is now free to stimulate her clit with one of her hands. This of course can be done with a vibrator or fingers.

Ease Of Position: Moderate

Intimacy Level: Moderate

Wild Spontaneous Level: High

Depth Of Penetration: Deep

Good For Female Orgasm? Yes

Downsides:

If the couple remains in this position for too long, her hips can become sore.

Upsides:

This position combines the vigor of bent over fucking with the ability for her to orgasm. This can create a very intense orgasm indeed.

Notes On This Position:

For the man, it is not a bad idea to slow down the penetration while she is building towards orgasm. If you fuck her too vigorously, you can impede the process. Remember, in this position your balls will be slapping into her clit region as well and that can cause an issue. More gentle fucking solves this problem and won't crash your balls onto her hand.

The man can also take over the clitoral stimulation. This can be a bit to juggle all at once, but using a vibrator will simplify things. Doing so will allow her to close her eyes and just be overwhelmed by the sensations and excitement.

The Reclining X

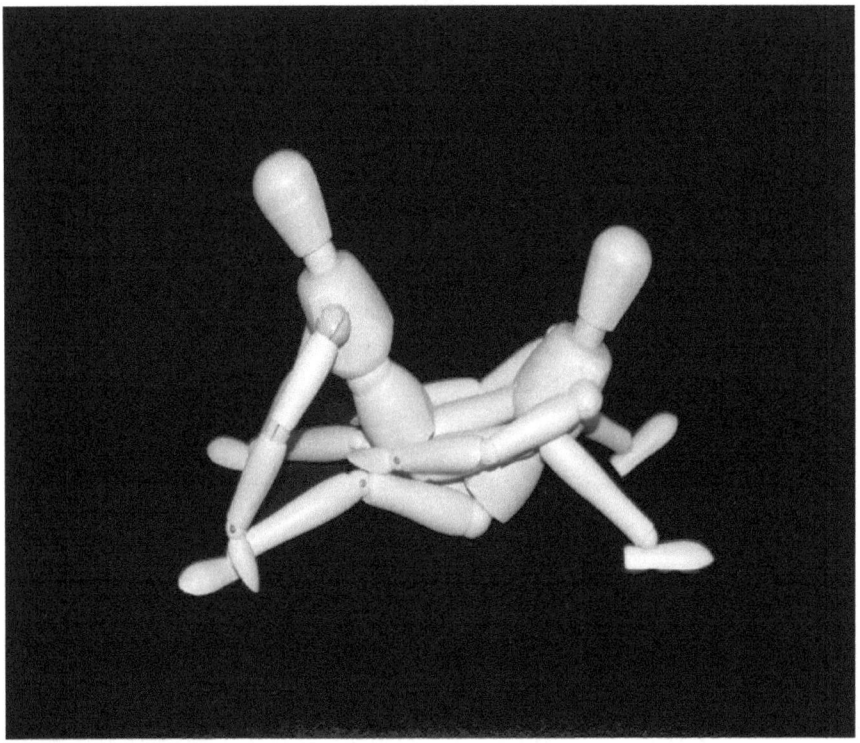

Position Description:

This position is best entered into from the "Cowgirl" position.

From the "Cowgirl" position, the woman leans back with her lover still inside of her. He sits up and places his hands on her lower back to support her as she shifts her weight. She brings her feet forward in front of her. He brings up his knees. She will now naturally slide down further onto his penis.

Ease Of Position: Moderate

Intimacy Level: High

Wild Spontaneous Level: Moderate

Depth Of Penetration: Deep

Good For Female Orgasm? No

Downsides:

The downside of this position is that it can be difficult to get into. The couple must work together as a team. It is easy for his cock to slide out of her as they are moving around. It is best to take it slow to make sure that this does not happen.

Upsides:

This position is very intimate. The two of you are facing each other as you are making love and this intensifies the bond. Penetration is deep and the two of you are very much physically connected as well.

There is more than enough visual stimulation to go around on this one as well. From the man's point of view he is actually able to see his cock going in and out of his lover. This will be a huge turn on to him and will make this seem like a wild sex position. Trust me. He will love seeing the penetration.

Notes On This Position:

This position is a real work out for both partners, as well as a good exercise in teamwork. Both of you will be in a position to move thanks to the fact that both of your knees are cocked. This means tat penetration can get very vigorous. Both of you can easily increase the intensity. You will need to work together to achieve this. This can involve talking during the act, which always helps to bring a couple together.

Guys, keep your hands on the small of her back or her ass. This will help to support her and make her part of the thrusting easier. This will also help keep you in the seated position. Ladies, you should use your hands to brace yourselves in the seated position. Use your legs and hips to do the actual fucking.

Although I put that this position is not good for female orgasm, that is not entirely true. During actual intercourse with him sliding in and out of her, there is really too much going on for clitoral stimulation to be reasonable. This is true. However, if the two of you stop the intercourse and just hold this position (no in and out) this position is actually very practical for female orgasm, especially with a vibrator. The fact that her hands are immobilized holding her up and he must make her cum, will actually be a turn on to a lot of women.

Missionary With Self Gratification

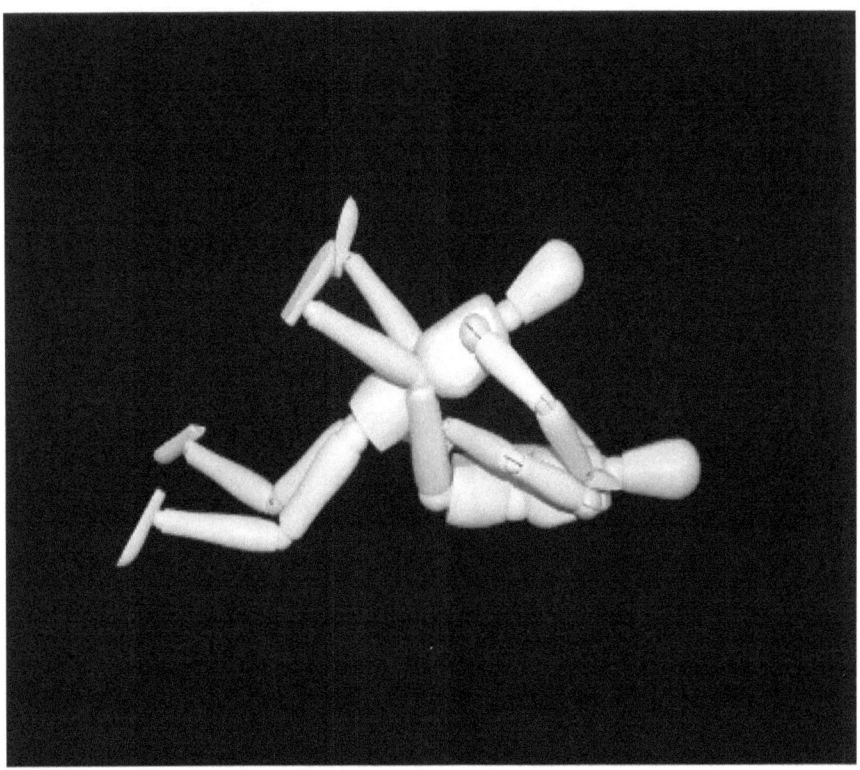

Position Description:

This position is a modification of the basic missionary position. In this position, the woman lies on her back and spreads her legs. The man lies between her legs and penetrates her. However, unlike in the basic missionary position, he does not extend his legs fully or lie flush on top of her.

Instead, with this position, he rests his weight on his knees, his pelvis and his hands and tilts his pelvis and penetration back. This exposes her clitoris. In this way she is able to stimulate her clitoris either through direct manual stimulation or a small vibrator.

Ease Of Position: Easy

Intimacy Level: High

Wild Spontaneous Level: Moderate

Depth Of Penetration: Below Average

Good For Female Orgasm? Yes

Downsides:

This position does not really have any downsides.

Upsides:

This position is a really good one to work into a couple's sexual repertoire. Both partners are in a position to orgasm and the possibility of simultaneous orgasm is high. The face to face contact also helps to build intimacy and bring the couple closer together.

Notes On This Position:

With this position, the man should try to limit his penetration. Going balls deep here can be counterproductive if she is using a vibrator. The space created by tilting back the pelvis is useful, but small. Full penetration may hit her hand or sex toy and in turn hit the clitoris. This painful for her and is to be avoided. However, this small detail is more than made up for the by the face to face intimacy that will enhance sexual pleasure for both partners.

As far as a position for female orgasm, this is one of the trickier ones and does require the couple to be in tune with each other, but it is definitely easy for a woman to orgasm in this position.

Cowgirl Lunge

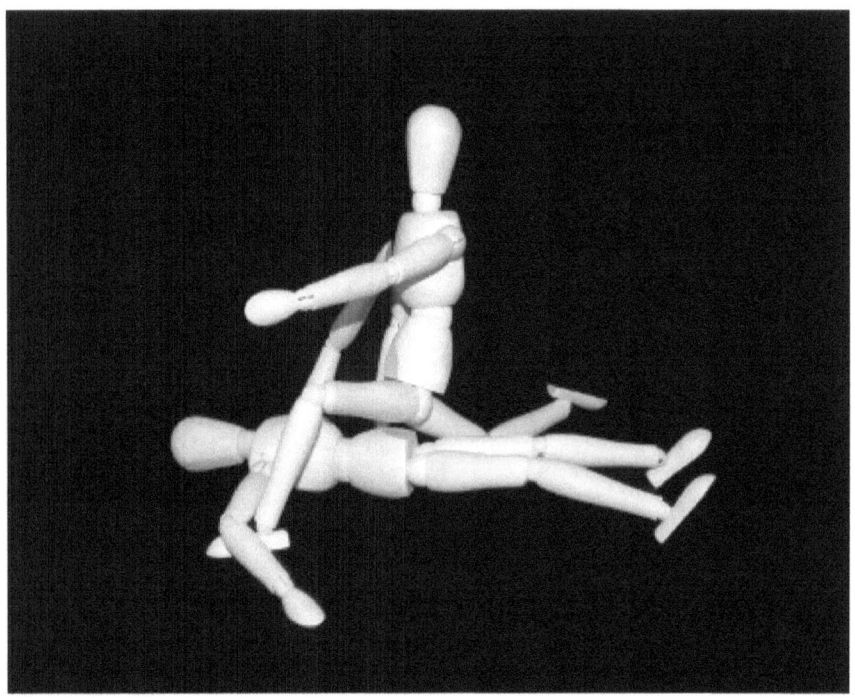

Position Description:

In the Cowgirl Lunge, the man lies on his back face up. The woman then straddles him with her weight resting on one of her knees. Her other leg is in the lunging position with her foot flush on the floor or bed. She then inserts his penis and rides it, like a cowgirl.

Ease Of Position: Difficult

Intimacy Level: Low

Wild Spontaneous Level: High

Depth Of Penetration: Deep

Good For Female Orgasm? Possible, but difficult

Downsides:

This position is not entirely stable for the woman and she will need to maintain balance the whole time. This can take away from her surrendering to the moment. Also, if she becomes overstimulated, she may easily loose her balance. This act should only be performed in a safe, soft area should she loose balance.

This position is also physically demanding and she may tire quickly.

Upsides:

This position offers her a great deal of control. She is able to use her leg muscles to really bounce up and down on his cock to her heart's delight. Also, by spreading her legs so wide, she is able to accommodate his whole body between her legs. This creates a nice flush contact between cock and pussy. She is able to go as deep as possible with penetration and using her leg muscles she is able to control how hard she is penetrated.

Notes On This Position:

This is a really wild position. She can really fuck her partner and herself in this position. Penetration can be hard, fast and deep and she is in total control. This can be a turn on to many men who will enjoy seeing their lover filled with such enthusiasm and passion.

This position also exposes her clitoris to stimulation. The only problem with actually stimulating it is that she tend to be bouncing up and down a lot and needs her hands to help her balance. There is, on the other hand, nothing wrong with pausing while he is still inside you to play with your clit to orgasm. It should be you that stimulates it in this position. He is not at the right angle to do it effectively or tenderly.

Bouncy Girl

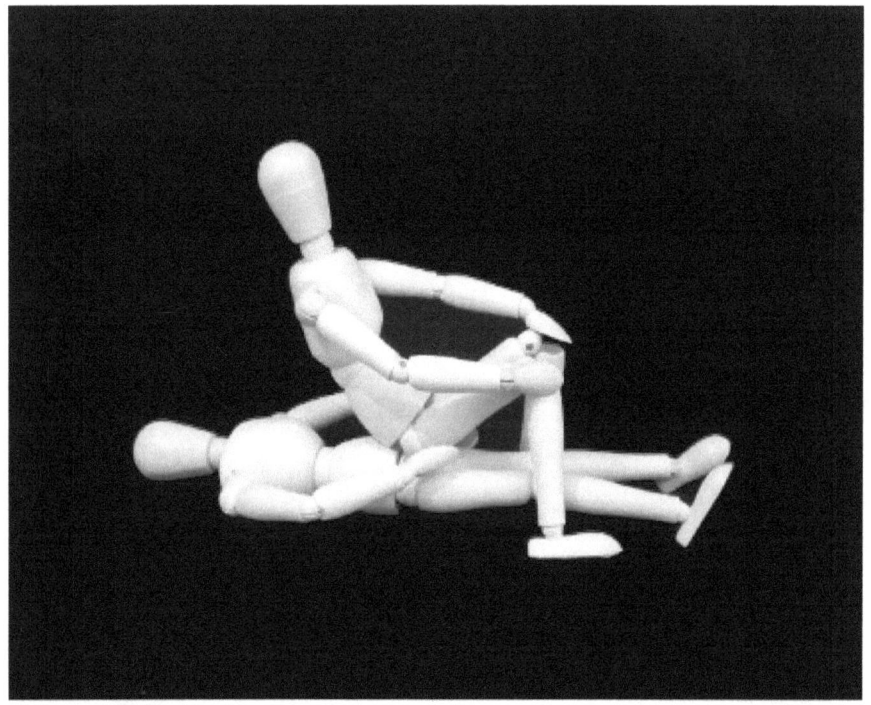

Position Description:

In the Bouncy Girl position, again the man starts by lying on his back with his erect penis pointing up. She then straddles him facing away from him and puts him inside her. Once he is inside her, she brings her feet up and places her weight on her soles. Her feet should be on either side of his legs. Her hands should rest on her knees.

She is now in a position to bounce up and down on his cock using her leg muscles and knees as leverage. The man can help to stabilize his lover as well as participate by placing his hands under her ass. Then, he can actually help lift her up and down. This will lower the amount of energy she needs to exert and will help prolong the act.

Ease Of Position: Moderate

Intimacy Level: Moderate

Wild Spontaneous Level: High

Depth Of Penetration: Moderate

Good For Female Orgasm? Impractical

Downsides:

There are no significant downsides to this position.

Upsides:

Upsides to this position are that she is in control of both speed and depth of penetration. This position is also less physically demanding than the cowgirl lunge and you can perform this act for a longer period of time.

Notes On This Position:

This position is a lot of fun. She is in control of penetration both in terms of speed and depth. However, there is a lot of action as she is literally bouncing up and down on his cock. Penetration is lower with this one because his cock is passing between her butt cheeks. This means that some of his penis is not actually going inside her. This can be good as in "woman on top" positions, sometimes the increased depth of penetration can cause cervical discomfort. This position reduces, if not eliminates this problem. Also, since she is resting on her butt cheeks, there is a higher lever of comfort.

\

<u>One Leg Over The Shoulder Missionary</u>

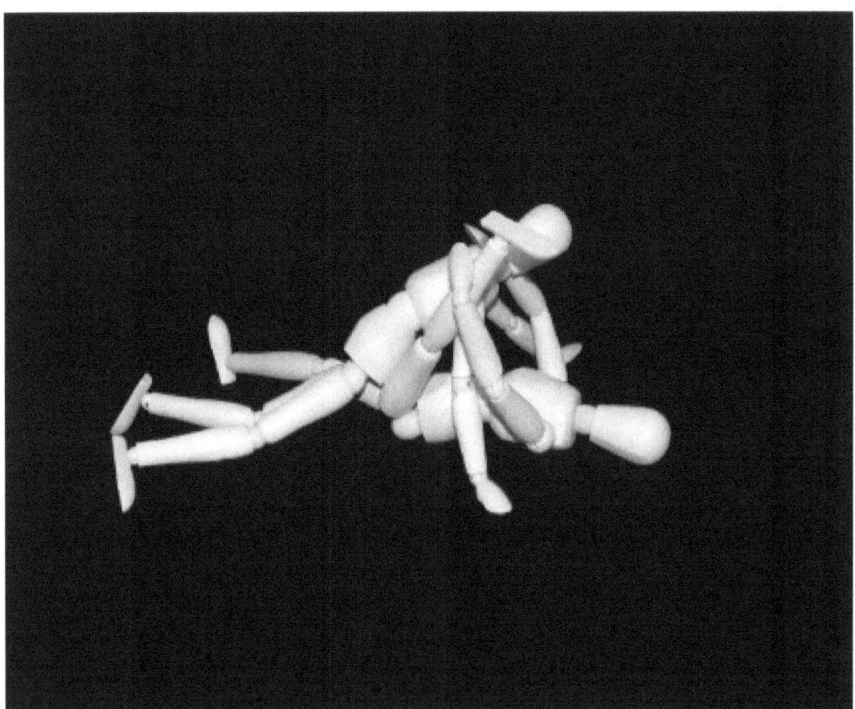

Position Description:

This position is a deeper penetration adaption of the
missionary position.

In this position, the woman lies on the bed just as she would during regular missionary position sex. The man, likewise, lies on top of her and then enters her, just like in missionary. However, with this position, while the couple is engaged in intercourse, she lifts her leg over one of his shoulders. It can be the right or the left. The side is immaterial. He aids in this act by lifting with the arm of the shoulder she is throwing her leg over.

This has the effect of spreading her legs wider than they would normally go (although still comfortable). This allows for a very flush cock to pussy contact which allows for very deep penetration.

Ease Of Position: Moderate

Intimacy Level: Moderate

Wild Spontaneous Level: Moderate

Depth Of Penetration: Deep

Good For Female Orgasm? No

Downsides:

This position requires her to keep her legs spread wide. This can put pressure on her hips and her muscles may grow tired after a bit. Also, because this position needs to be entered into while intercourse is already happening without removal, his cock can slide out while you are making the transition. Not that big of a deal though.

Upsides:

The upsides of this position are deeper penetration, more vigorous lovemaking and face to face contact. This has the effect of increasing the bond between the couple and creating a very lively, very satisfying sexual experience.

Notes On This Position:

This position is average in all three categories of ease, wildness, and intimacy. This means that it is a solid, reliable position that should find a place in your regular sexual antics. It is enjoyable for both partners and feels great to both as well. Just keep in mind how long it has been going on to keep her hips from getting sore.

Reverse Cowgirl

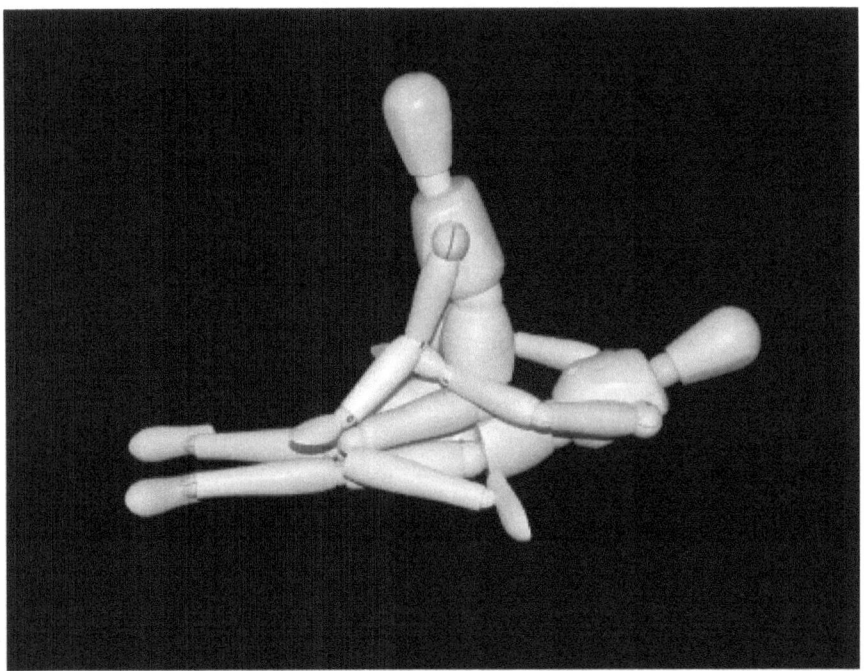

Position Description:

In Reverse Cowgirl the man lies down and the woman straddles him and sits down onto his cock, inserting it into her in the process. The difference between this position and Bouncy Girl is that in this position, her knees remain bent and her weight is borne by her shins.

This means that she is not lifting nearly as high with Reverse Cowgirl as she is with Bouncy Girl. This means that there is less friction, less vigorous penetration and there is less chance or any cervical discomfort.

Ease Of Position: Moderate

Intimacy Level: Low

Wild Spontaneous Level: Moderate

Depth Of Penetration: Average

Good For Female Orgasm? Yes

Downsides:

The Reverse Cowgirl has the disadvantage of being a position in which the woman is looking away from the man. There is no face to face contact. All she can see of him is his feet. This is similar to Doggystyle, but there are none of the domination aspects involved that make up for this problem in Doggystyle. She is in control, but can't even look her man in the face to make sure he knows it.

Upsides:

The upside for Reverse Cowgirl is that there is gentle penetration and good access to her clitoris. This means that she is in a great position to masturbate while her lover is inside her either manually or with a vibrator. The gentle penetration also means that he is not terribly likely to cum and go limp while she is doing this. The gentle penetration should keep him hard while she masturbates to her satisfaction.

Reverse Cowgirl also has the advantage that is very visually stimulating from the man's point of view. If she tilts her hips forward only slightly, her pussy, with his cock sliding slowly in and out of it is revealed. This is something any man would enjoy. If she tilts her hips forward and brings her shoulders and spine down as well, her whole vulva is on brilliant display for him. For him, this is a feast for the eyes he can't get enough.

Notes On This Position:

One trick with this position is keeping his cock from sliding out of her. The angle of her vagina is not especially conducive to this position with fast penetration. Most likely he will slip out. If this does happen, it is easy enough to reinsert him, and continue.

Another note on this position is that with her leaning forward, her ass is right there for him to see. To some women, this may cause a bit of bashfulness. For others who enjoy having their asses stimulated, this is a positive. One way or the other, most men, especially young men, will have trouble resisting such a lovely bit of temptation. He may choose to try and stimulate you whether or not you have made it clear that you enjoy that. It's best to have a conversation beforehand.

Doggystyle Reach Around

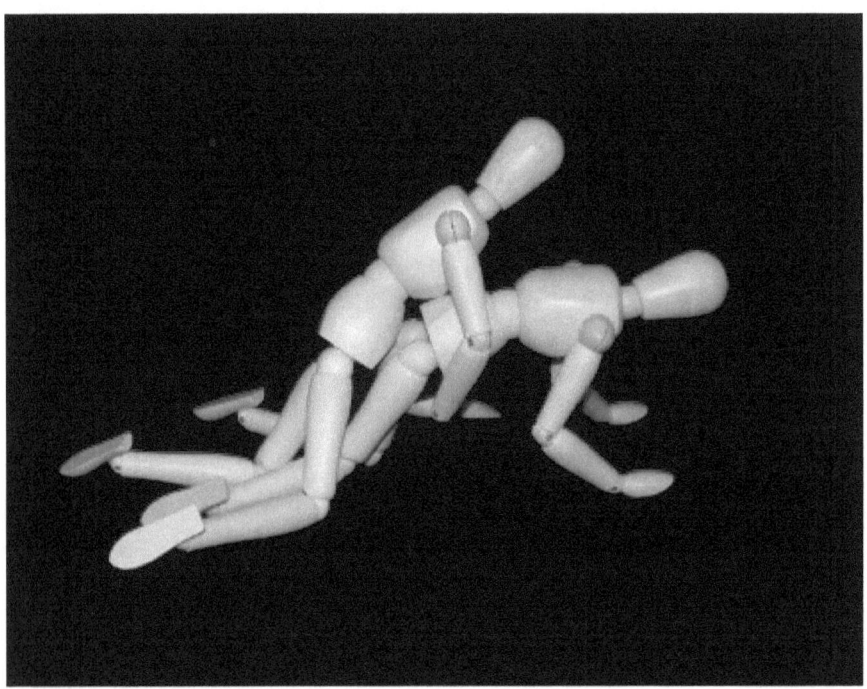

Position Description:

This is a modification of the doggystyle position. In this incarnation, the couple assumes the usual doggystyle position. However there are two differences.

The first is that the woman can move her legs outside of the man's. This will give her the ability to widen her legs to their full extent.

The second modification is that the man reaches under the woman's tummy down to her clitoris. Here, in this position, he is able to stimulate her clitoris with either a vibrator or his fingers.

Ease Of Position: Easy

Intimacy Level: High

Wild Spontaneous Level: High

Depth Of Penetration: Deep

Good For Female Orgasm? Yes

Downsides:

Like any position that has the man involved in actual penetration at the same time he is stimulating the woman's clitoris, he can get too rough. Often he does not realize just how sensitive her clitoris is and he can apply too much friction and pressure with the best of intentions. It is important that he understand that he should start very lightly and only then slowly increase. He should also pay special attention to her body movements as the act continues. If she is enjoying it, she will make it known very quickly.

Now ladies, this warning does not absolve you of any responsibility. You need to make sure that you are communicating with your partner. Tell him when it feels good and what he needs to do. Men appreciate and desire your help very badly!

Upsides:

This position combines deep penetration with clitoral stimulation. This is huge. It is one thing for a woman to cum while he is eating her pussy. Cumming while getting fucked is a whole different world. This position should definitely have a place in your bedroom fun.

Notes On This Position:

This position is high on intimacy and wild spontaneity. Not many positions in this book can make that same claim. In most cases, you trade one for the other. This is a definite exception. Yes, the couple is not facing one another and that takes away from the intimacy. However, he is making an effort to make her have an orgasm for a change. This makes her feel cared for, respected and appreciated. These are huge and more than make up for the lack of eye contact.

This position has a lot of pluses going for it and it should be in your tool box, however, you need to make sure that you talk about this act before just going for it. I am definitely talking to the guys here. Don't just surprise her. Let her know that you want to do this and work at it together. There is some coordination that needs to be worked out, but any couple with good communication skills can quickly master these challenges.

Doggystyle Self Gratification

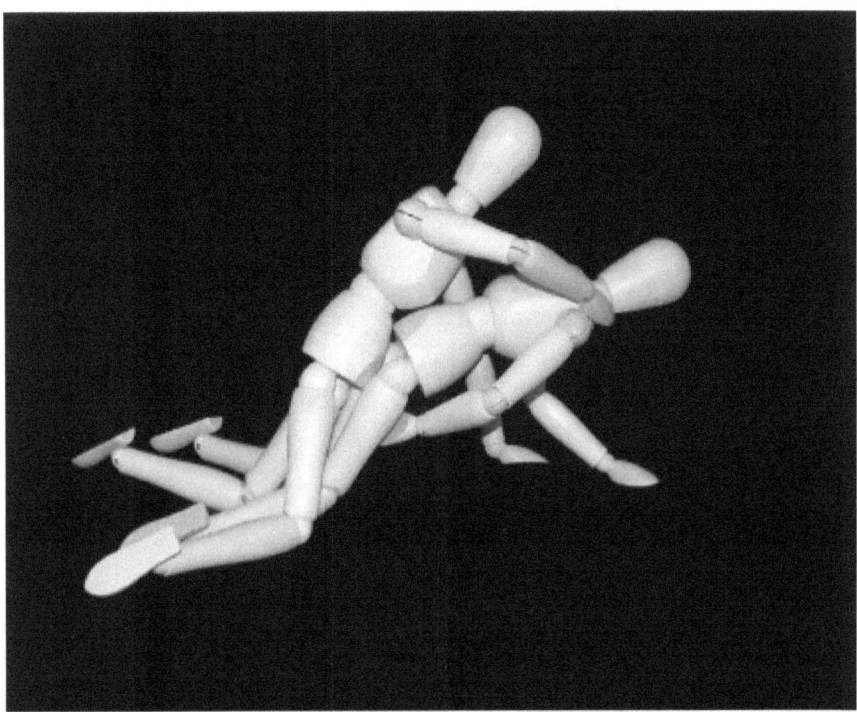

Position Description:

This position is yet another incarnation of the doggystyle. Just like the regular doggystyle, the woman gets on all fours and the man enters her from behind. However, in this position, instead of the man, the woman stimulates her own clitoris to orgasm.

Ease Of Position: Easy

Intimacy Level: Moderate

Wild Spontaneous Level: Moderate

Depth Of Penetration: Deep

Good For Female Orgasm? Yes

Downsides:

With one hand on her clitoris, the woman is in a less stable position. The man will often put his wieght on her shoulders while he is fucking her. This can result in an unstable situation and the couple can collapse. To avoid this, the man should keep his weight on his legs and off of her altogether.

Upsides:

With her in control of the stimulation to her clit, she is in total control of her orgasm. He will not get too rough and chafe her. Also, she is in the position to give herself a powerful orgasm while he is inside of her. This combination is a definite plus to any couple's sex repertoire and one that is all too often elusive. Every couple should give it a try.

Notes On This Position:

In this position, if the man is fucking away, he can easily interfere with her finger or vibrator stimulation. This is especially true if she has a vibrator on her clit. He can easily hit it and jam it into her clit. Again, this is painful to say the least.

While she is pleasuring herself the man should not concentrate on sliding in and out of her pussy. Instead, it is better for him to insert himself balls deep and then apply gentle pressure into her vagina with his hips. If he is doing this correctly, he will give her the sensation of vigorous penetration without his penis moving in and out of her at all. This technique will also slow down his orgasm and allow her to finish hers. This position is more about her orgasm than his.

Once she has climaxed to her satisfaction, the couple can resume normal doggystyle until he has orgasmed as well.

Bend Her Over Something

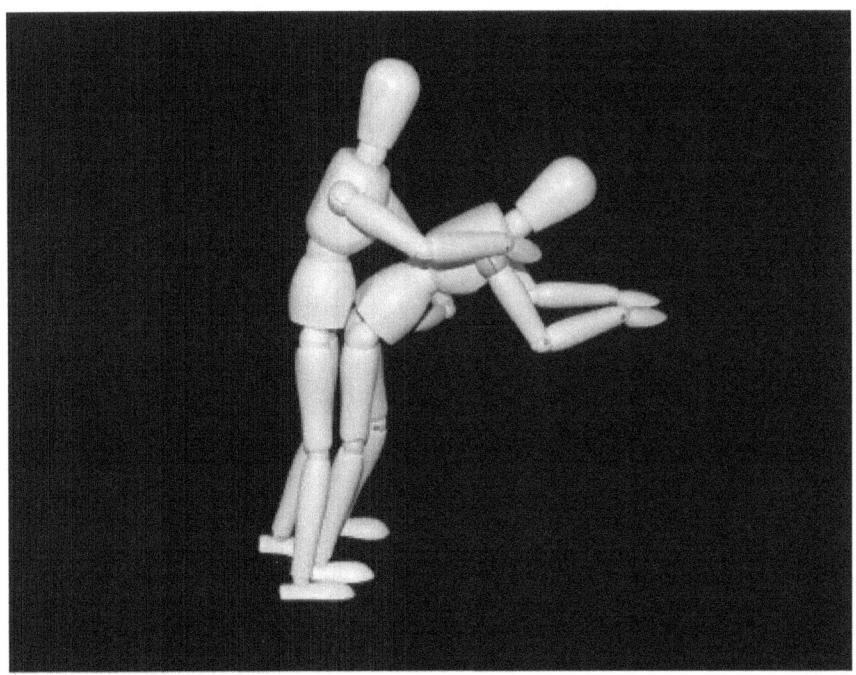

Position Description:

This position is simple. The woman bends over something
(table, counter top, bed, hood of a car) from the standing
position. She spreads her ankles shoulder width apart. This
offers access to her pussy and ass. The man then approaches
her from behind. He enters her in this way and sex
commences.

Ease Of Position: Easy

Intimacy Level: Low

Wild Spontaneous Level: High

Depth Of Penetration: Deep

Good For Female Orgasm? No

Downsides:

This position is low on intimacy. In fact, this position is the one so often featured in prison rape scenes in movies. Now that is not to say that this position is violent, unloving or inappropriate for affectionate lovers. Far from it. Sometimes a woman really just wants to get bent over and fucked and her man friend is usually more than enthusiastic.

All that being said, this should not necessarily be your first "go to" position. This should be a position that is engaged in in the heat of passion. It is always best to start out with some intimate, slower positions as a warm up and once the temperature has reached boiling point, then its time for someone to bend over and get wildly fucked - but only then.

Upsides:

This position offers a lot of dominance that is often enjoyed by both partners, like we've seen before. The man enter the woman in the dominant position and vigorously fucks her. The woman is able to enjoy the submissive role as well as the deep and vigorous penetration.

This position also has the advantage of expediency. It can be engaged in in limited space like a closet, shower, or even airplane bathroom. It is also capable to engage in this position while still fully clothed. All she needs to do is drop her pants and panties or lift her skirt and pull them to the side. He on the other hand can also drop his pants or can just unzip his fly.

On a side note, a gentleman always drops his pants when bending his woman over in a clothed position. Those metal teeth on your zipper can easily scuff her pussy or even her clit if you are pounding away vigorously.

Notes On This Position:

Due to the dominance issues that were just discussed, this position is appropriate for additional dominance play like spanking and hair pulling. As with common sexual practices that **can** be unwelcome (these, for example) it is always best for the couple to discuss these acts before intercourse. Nothing will ruin the mood of sex faster that a red hand print (playfully intended) on an unsuspecting woman's ass.

Bend Her Over Aristocratically

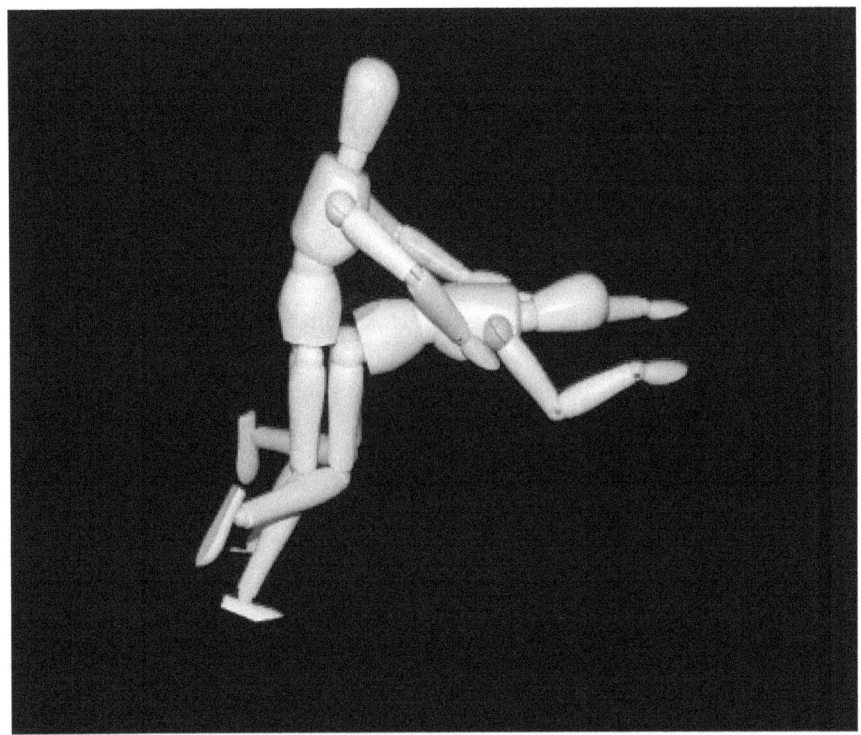

Position Description:

This position, like "Aristocratic Pussy eating" requires a soft piece of furniture. This too is a a sexual position for the living room.

She assumes a four point stance on the piece of furniture with her knees on the seat and her arms over the back. She can be nude, but since this is a great quickie position, she can just as easily hike her skirt or drop her pants exposing her pussy and ass.

He approaches her fro behind, perhaps from the "Aristocratic Pussyeating" position and penetrates her. He can penetrate her either vaginally or anally depending on the preference of the couple.

Ease Of Position: Easy

Intimacy Level: Moderate

Wild Spontaneous Level: High

Depth Of Penetration: Deep

Good For Female Orgasm? Yes

Downsides:

There are no appreciable downsides to this position. Her knees are comforted and the position is gentle on her body.

Upsides:

This position is dripping with wild sex and spontaneity. She's hiked her skirt, he's dropped his pants and the two of you are surfing waves of passion in the mid-afternoon, in the living room while the kids are at school.

Notes On This Position:

Just because you can go from "Aristocratic Pussyeating" to this position does not mean that you cannot go from this position to "Aristocratic Pussyeating". The two of you may not be able to control your lust and may be forced to strip half naked and plunge into sexual intercourse before you know what is happening. If so, well then bravo. Enjoy!

However, for the man, there is nothing wrong with fucking your woman for a while to bring the rosiness to her cheeks, and then dropping down to eat her pussy afterwards. If you are concerned about cum, fuck her for a while, then eat her pussy, then fuck her until you cum. In that situation, everyone wins! The two of you are sexually sated for a bit and you can get on with the day, maybe even go back to work and smile about what the two of you did on your lunch break.

Downward Doggystyle With Self Gratification

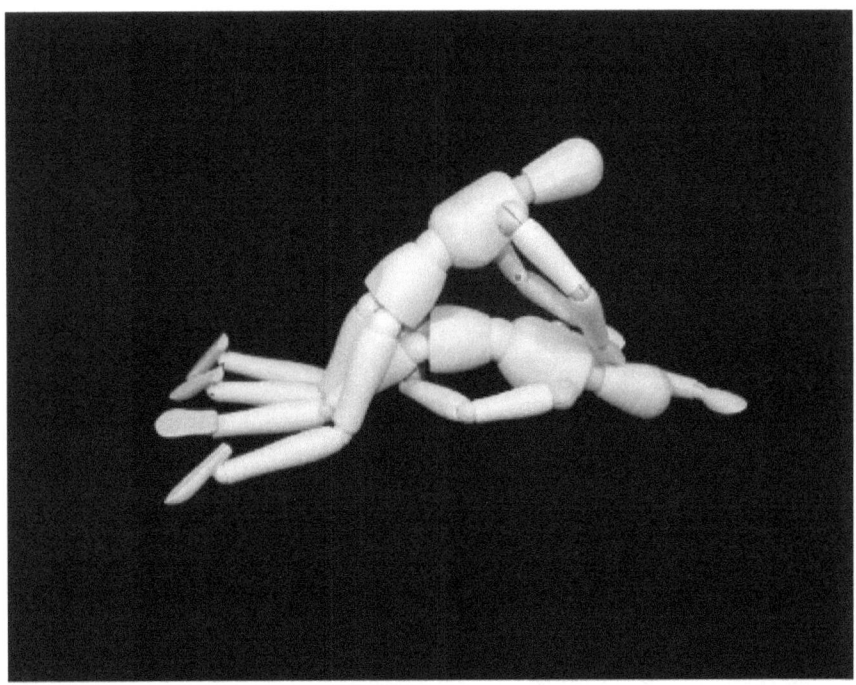

Position Description:

This is yet another modification of the "Doggystyle" position.

The couple begins with ordinary doggystyle. However, the woman relaxes and actually rests her face on the bed. This has two effects.

The first is that she elongates her back and and angles her vagina down allowing for deeper penetration. This can really make this position much hotter. The other is that, as she is no longer relying on her arms for support, they are now free to stimulate her clit and even play with his balls.

Ease Of Position: Easy

Intimacy Level: Moderate

Wild Spontaneous Level: Moderate

Depth Of Penetration: Deep

Good For Female Orgasm? Yes

Downsides:

Since she is face down on the bed, this can become uncomfortable after a bit. This also rules this position out on hard surfaces like a floor, unless a pillow is involved. Even on the bed, the pillows can be a big help. Make sure one is handy!

As the penetration is very deep, there can be some cervical discomfort after a time. It really all depends on her and her body.

Upsides:

There are a lot of pluses to this position. The penetration is about as deep as it can get. This is huge to many women.

There is also a domination factor. The man has her bent over, face down and is really giving it to her hard. This is a turn on for both partners. It would not be inappropriate to employ some playful hair pulling or ass slapping with this position either.

Notes On This Position:

This is the author's favorite incarnation of the "Doggystyle" position. She is playing with her clit while he is balls deep inside her vigorously fucking her. The sex is hot and vigorous. Don't try this position at home if the kids are there. Things will get hot and loud enough that they will wonder what is going on in the bedroom. Wait until you have some alone time.

Basic Doggystyle

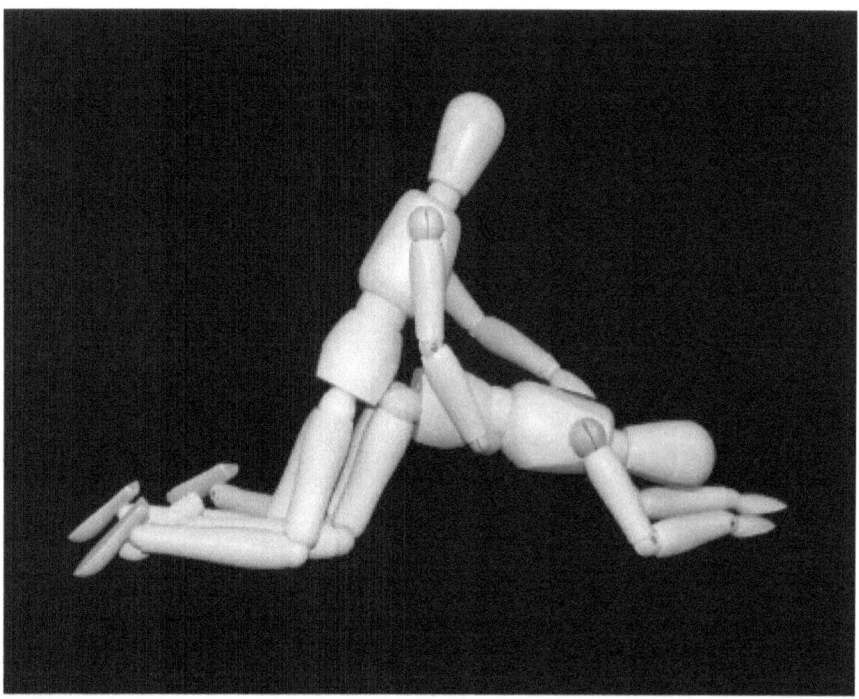

Position Description:

In this position, the woman assumes a four point stance on the bed, floor, or even couch. He then approaches her from behind and inserts himself into her. This can be good for both anal or vaginal intercourse.

Once the man is inside her, he can the buck his hips forward and back as he slides in and out of her.   Her butt cheeks will act as a cushion so he can fuck her more vigorously than otherwise would be possible.

If she wants she can lower her head and shoulders at the same time she arches her back. This will actually expose her pussy to deeper penetration. By making adjustments, she can find the depth that is just right for her.

Ease Of Position: Easy

Intimacy Level: Low

Wild Spontaneous Level: High

Depth Of Penetration: Deep

Good For Female Orgasm? No

Downsides:

The only downside with this position is that there is no face to face time. This means no eye contact, less emotional connection and no kissing. (He can kiss all over her neck and back.) This can definitely take away from this position's desirability. That is not to say that this position should no have no place in your lovemaking. On the contrary, this position is a lot of fun, just make sure that this is not the only way you ever make love. Switch it up from this, to something more intimate, like "Basic Missionary".

Upsides:

This is a wild position. The sex tends to be more vigorous, and more passionate. This is one of those positions that a couple will assume when they both just want to fuck each other. The penetration is deeper and more forceful. Also, the woman will often enjoy this position because she feels that the man is in control. It is not at all uncommon or weird for a woman to enjoy some hair pulling and ass slapping as she gets fucked in this position. As always with rougher sex, talk about it first.

Notes On This Position:

In this position, like with all Doggystyle variants, her ass is right there tempting her lover. He most likely will give thought to playing with it, maybe even doing some inserting. Well, this should never happen without her advanced permission, or decent lubrication. Anal should always be a decision reached in advance by the couple. Of course her saying "Stick a finger in may ass." does count, but the man should wait until there is an obvious green light. Never just assume with anal!

It is also important to point out that the man is not the only one who can do the fucking in this position. The woman can definitely get in on the action by moving her body forward and back on her knees. She can even do this in time with his motions. This will cause a rough impact when the two come together and can really make for some rough, deep impact sex if that is what the couple is looking for.

Double Handed Buttlift

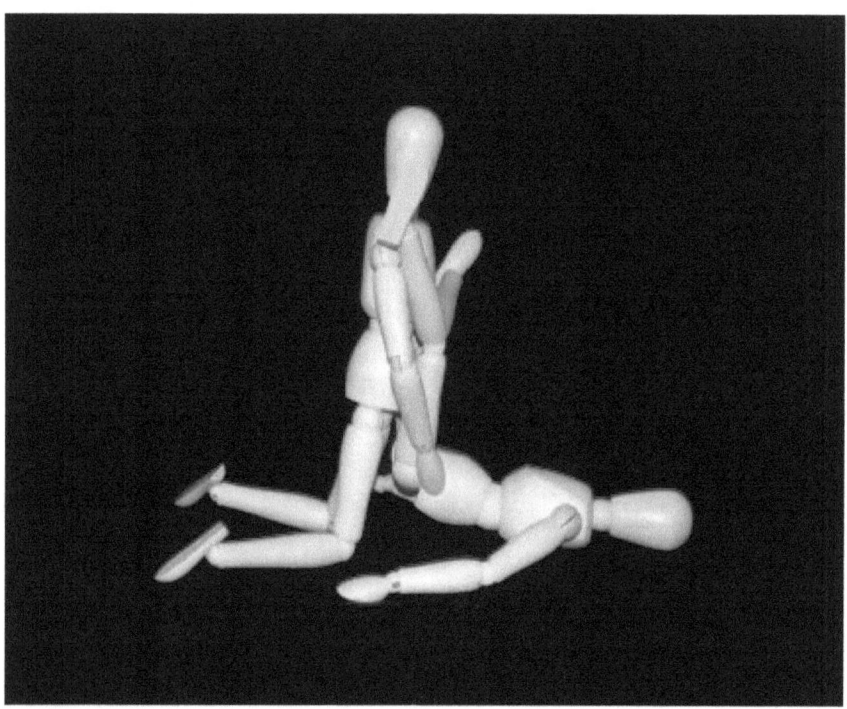

Position Description:

This position is assumed from the missionary position once penetration has occurred. Also, penetration is not interrupted as you go into this position.

From the missionary position, he takes her legs and throws both of them over his shoulder. With an ankle on either side of his head, he can now reach down and firmly grab an ass cheek with each hand and lift her up.

This will allow for much deeper penetration, and usually more vigorous penetration as well.

Ease Of Position: Moderate

Intimacy Level: Moderate

Wild Spontaneous Level: High

Depth Of Penetration: Deep

Good For Female Orgasm? No

Downsides:

This position place some strains on the man's back. He is bearing a lot more weight than he normally does. This can be a problem.

Upsides:

This position allows for the deep penetration of "Doggystyle" with the face to face contact of the "Missionary" position. This is a very positive combination that will make the position a plus to both partners.

This position also put the man firmly in the dominant role once again. This can be a plus for women who want the man to take control in the bedroom as well.

Notes On This Position:

In this position, the woman's feet are right up by the man's face. This is an opportunity that should not be missed! A secret that too many couples overlook is that women love to have attention paid to their feet. It feels even better when they are having sex. I mean that the man should kiss all over her feet and suck and lick her toes until she coos with delight. Trust me, she will.

Basic Missionary

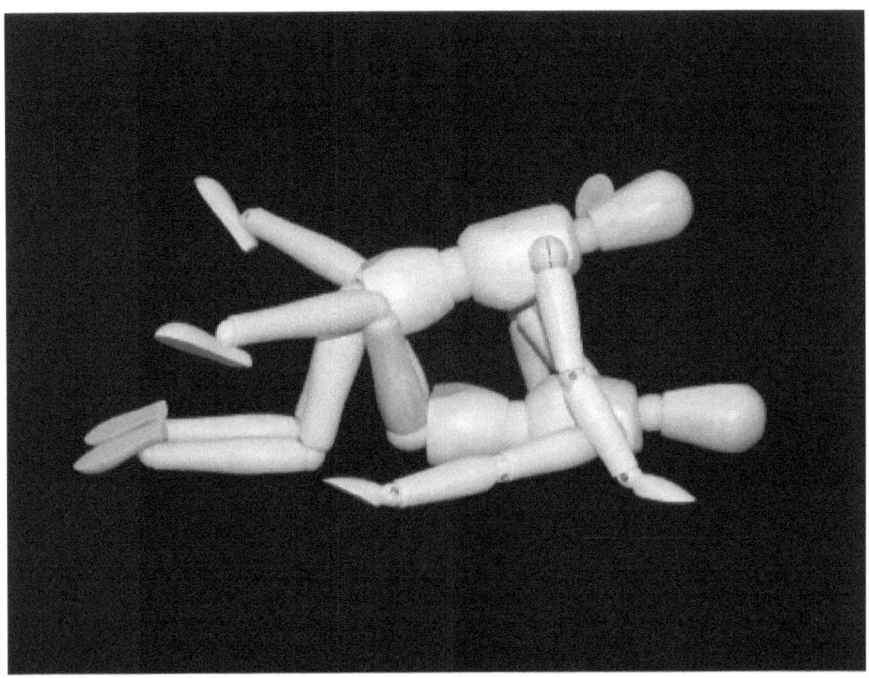

Position Description:

In the Basic missionary position, the woman lies on the bed or floor. She bends her knees and firmly plants her feet. Her lover, then lies between her legs and penetrates her. He moves his hips so his cock moves in and out of her. For her comfort, the woman can lift her feet and place them around the back of her lover.

Although not a basic requirement of this position there should be lots of kissing, nuzzling, licking, nibbling and whispering of sweet nothings between the couple. The closeness is one of the biggest pluses of this position.

Ease Of Position: Easy

Intimacy Level: High

Wild Spontaneous Level: Low

Depth Of Penetration: Average

Good For Female Orgasm? No

Downsides:

There is no downside to this position. Anyone can do it. It's comfortable and you can make love by the fire using this position all night.

Upsides:

This is a very tender and intimate position. You should use it to do just that. It makes a great position when penetration first occurs, after foreplay. Think of it as a warm up position.

This position is also a great one for first time sex.

Notes On This Position:

This position has a bit of a reputation for being boring. People think of it as plain old vanilla sex. Although this position is a tried and true one, the reputation for boring is a bit undeserved.

instead of boring, you should look at this position as one of the most intimate positions in this book. There is so much that is going on here that builds closeness between lovers. There is face to face contact. The whole of your body is pressed to your lovers. You can feel each others warmth, and if the sex is slow and tender, even heartbeats. There should always be lots of kissing. By this I mean all over the neck, breasts, cheeks, earlobes and of course lips.

This is also not to say that this position cannot take on a "dirtier" persona. This is the position in which men earn scratches on their backs too! Think of this as a sexual position with a speed setting. In slow, it is tender, loving and intimate. In high, it is a back scratching ride through ecstasy and passion. This is why is THE classic sex position.

Cowgirl Up

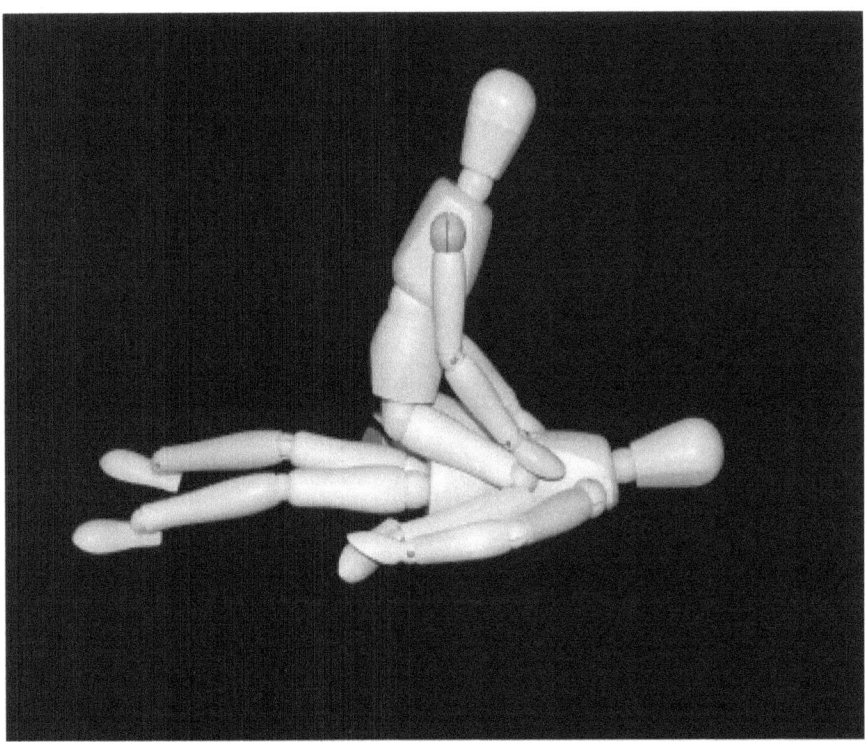

Position Description:

In this position, the man lies on the bed and the woman mounts him facing him. She inserts his cock into her and then rests on it in the seated position.

She is not firmly in control of the intercourse. She can rock her hips forward gently for subtle vaginal stimulation. If she chooses to she can also bounce more vigorously on his cock using her leg muscles.

Ease Of Position: Easy

Intimacy Level: High

Wild Spontaneous Level: Moderate

Depth Of Penetration: Deep

Good For Female Orgasm? Honestly...debatable

Downsides:

There are no downsides to this position. It is easy and fun for all involved.

Upsides:

The woman is firmly in control of the action here. It's her turn to be dominant. This is a thrill for many women and a chance for them to take over and really fuck their partner for a change.

This position is versatile. If the couple wants to hold hands and look each other in the eye, they are connected and close. If, on the other hand, she wants to hold his wrists to the bed and fuck the hell out of him, she is capable of that as well. Again, think of this position as having a variable speed setting.

Notes On This Position:

As was mentioned, this position is versatile. There are two things that a couple should always try out. First, if the couple locks fingers and holds hands, he can support her while she vigorously fucks him. This will help her with support and he can even help lift her through her hands.

Also, the image demonstrating this position shows the woman in the upright position. This is for demonstration purposes only. She has the full range of motion and can come down and make out with her lover as well. By doing this she can increase the intimacy and even take a load of weight off her back. This position is also a great resting position after some wild monkey sex. It's great for a breather without interrupting the sex.

Now there is some debate about this position, as far as female orgasm goes that should be made clear here. First of all, her clitoris is not in a good location to be stimulated in this position. Her pubic bone is in the way. However, there are some other options that can be tried.

In this position, his cock will naturally apply pressure to the front inside wall of her vagina. Also, her clitoris is being pressed down on by her weight against his body. By manipulating this combination of factors, many women (empirically speaking) have been able to achieve orgasm in this position.

Now, this is not the kind of thing that will happen instantly. The woman has to be good and turned on and relaxed (just like oral sex). Lots of foreplay helps tremendously. She must also be able to keep all of her body movements coordinated as she approaches orgasm.

If the couple wishes to experiment with this (and they should), have the man lie on the bed and stay still. Guys, I know you want to move, but for her sake, just lay there and let her play with riding your cock. I know it's hard, but if she cums, it will be worth it. Have some fun with it. See what works. Giggle together and enjoy yourselves. Who knows, you may find a way for her to cum in this position and that is always something to celebrate.

Seated Face To Face Embrace

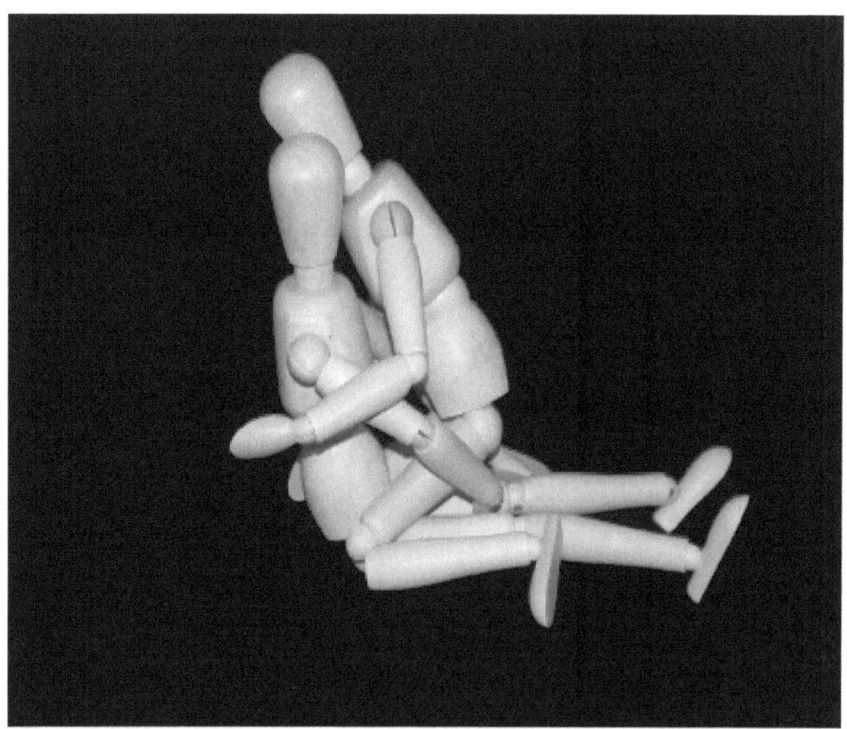

Position Description:

This position starts out in the "Cowgirl Up" position.
However, there is a twist.

The man sits up to meet and embrace the woman. He can also prop himself against a wall or pillows for comfort.

Ease Of Position: Easy

Intimacy Level: High

Wild Spontaneous Level: Low

Depth Of Penetration: Deep

Good For Female Orgasm? No

Downsides:

In this position, penetration and thrusting are limited by the close proximity of the lovers. Any movement is most likely going to come from her. She is in a position to use her hips and legs to lift her and then come back down. This can be tiring after a bit.

Upsides:

This position is as intimate as "Missionary". The lovers are very close and are holding one another. They are face to face so there should be lots of kissing on the lips, neck and breasts. This works to bring the lovers together.

Notes On This Position:

This is another position that does not require a lot of exertion by either of the partners to keep things going. As such you should consider this another resting position that is good when you need to catch your breath.

Crisscross

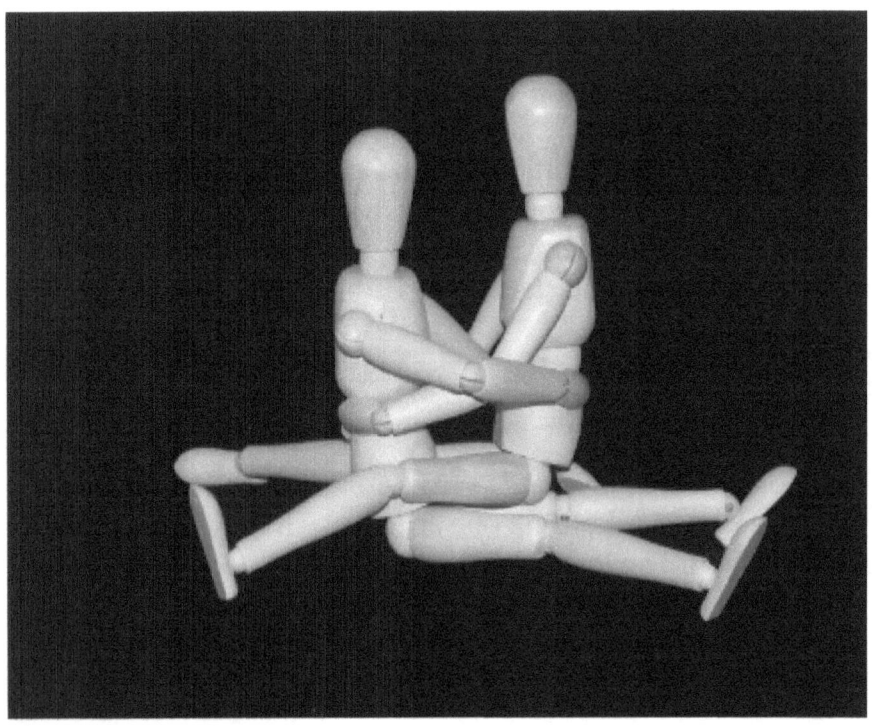

Position Description:

In this position, the man sits on the bed or floor with his back perpendicular to his legs. His legs are fully extended. She sits down on his penis and inserts it into her. Her legs should be on either side of him. She is resting her weight on his thighs. If one were to look down on the couple from above, their legs should form an "X".

Once she is seated on his thighs and his cock is comfortable inside her, the couple can adjust their legs for comfort. The couple can then rock their hips for mutual pleasure.

Ease Of Position: Easy

Intimacy Level: High

Wild Spontaneous Level: Low

Depth Of Penetration: Deep

Good For Female Orgasm? No

Downsides:

In this position, the couple has almost no range of motion beyond simply rocking hips. Now, this can feel great, however, this type of stimulation is unlikely to result in orgasm for either partner. This position is really best for the closeness it affords.

Upsides:

This position is amazingly intimate. You are flush with your partner. At times you are so close you can feel each others heartbeat and breathing rythem. There is a true oneness for the couple that comes from this position.

Notes On This Position:

This position is a great resting position. There is not a lot of work that is needed to be done by either partner. However, there is just enough movement to keep pussies wet and cocks hard. So, after you have been vigorously taking turns fucking each other for the better part of the last hour, you can rely on this position to catch your breath.

This position also affords the couple some serious face to face make out time that it would be foolish to ignore. You're right there staring at each other, so what better to do than make out...a lot. This is one of the best things going for this position. You can kiss all you want while your body takes a rest. Your spirits revive and you feel deeply connected to your lover, from either point of view.

Secretary On The Desk

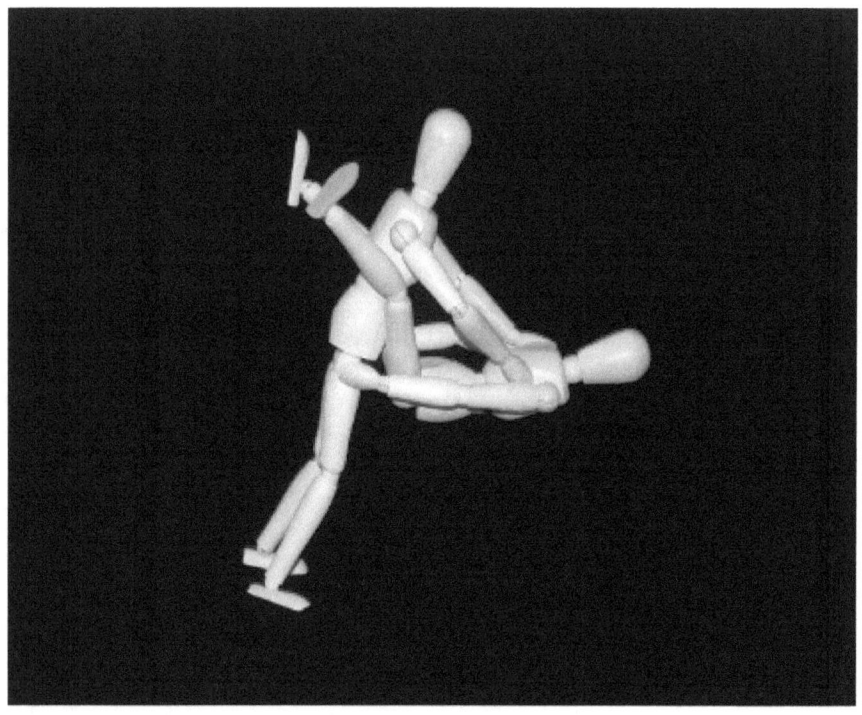

Position Description:

The "Secretary On The Desk" position is a variant on the "Missionary" sexual position.

In this position, the woman lies on a raised surface that is sufficiently high enough to allow the man to penetrate her while he is still in the standing position. Some examples of sufficiently high surfaces include an office desk, a pool table, car trunk or hood, or dining room table.

Ease Of Position: Easy

Intimacy Level: Moderate

Wild Spontaneous Level: High

Depth Of Penetration: Average

Good For Female Orgasm? No

Downsides:

One big downside to this position is that the woman is usually lying on a hard surface. This can limit her comfort during the sexual act.

Upsides:

This position can be assumed in many places. This makes it a very versatile position. Along with the fact that, provided the woman is wearing a skirt, no undressing is needed. I have heard tales of women taking their panties off in a restaurant and seeing if the bathroom changing tables can support the weight of them and their lovers.

Notes On This Position:

I will start by saying that this position is a lot of fun. When two people engage in this activity, there is a high level of passion. The two of you cannot wait to melt into one another tender embrace and are often forced to sweep everything on the table or desk onto the floor. Skirt hiking, passionate, vigorous lovemaking usually follows.

This position is also versatile in that you can engage in it either as preliminary sex or it can be the entire act. If it is preliminary sex, the two of you can't wait to begin. You fuck a little to tide you over while you move somewhere more comfortable. If this is the case, you are usually in for a long night of passion. If, on the other hand, this is the whole sex act, it will usually be brief. "I haven't seen you in six months sex" qualifies. The two of you fuck for a minute or two and the man quickly cums. If this is the case, most likely you will be recharged in a few minutes and be ready for more.

<u>Side By Side</u>

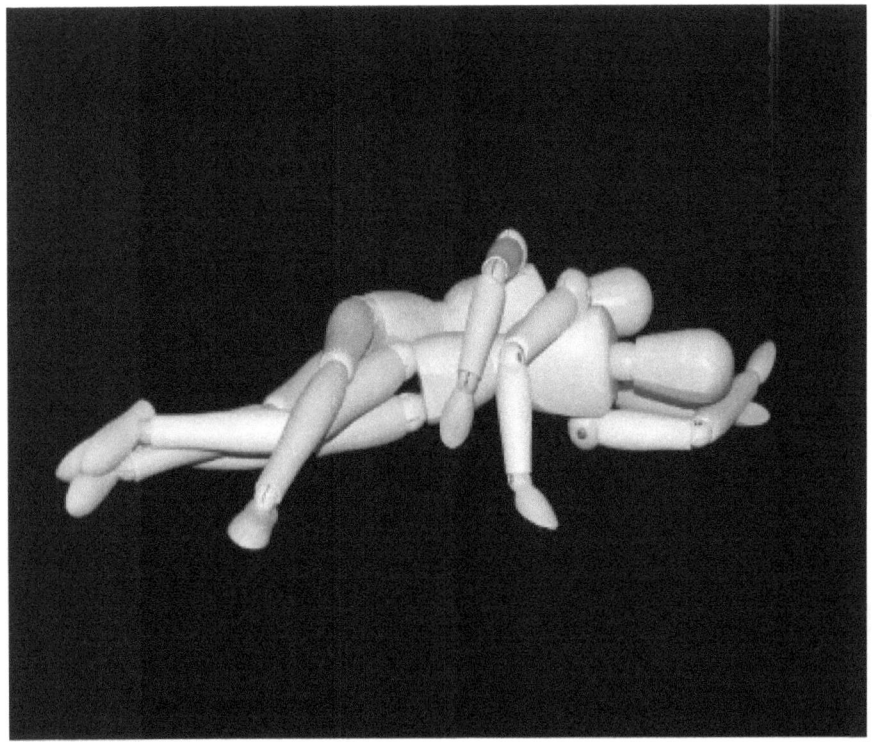

Position Description:

In this position, the woman lies on the bed and the man lies behind her, in a spooning position. She bends forward, as though she was being bent over (just on her side). This will make it easier for him to penetrate her. He inserts himself into her and commences lovemaking.

At this point, she can straighten her body to be close to him, or she can remain in a bent manner to allow for deeper penetration.

Ease Of Position: Easy

Intimacy Level: High

Wild Spontaneous Level: Low

Depth Of Penetration: Average

Good For Female Orgasm? No

Downsides:

This position is one that used for gentle, tender lovemaking. If the couple is looking for more vigorous and deep penetration, the should consider another position. Other than that, this position has no downsides.

Upsides:

This is a slow restful position. Since both partner's bodies are being supported by the bed, neither has to use their muscles to keep themselves upright. No one will fall over either, like in some of the more complicated positions. This position can be used as a rest position once the couple has grown tired, but still wants to continue having sex.

Notes On This Position:

As was said, this position is good as a resting position. It is also the best position for morning sex. If the partners have slept together it is easy to start spooning, get a little horny, and just slip right into this position. That way even morning breath can't stop the action.

This is also still a very intimate position even though it is not face to face. The lovers bodies are in full contact with each other. There are lots of opportunity for hip grabbing and breast cupping as well. Hands can roam and backs of necks should definitely be kissed!

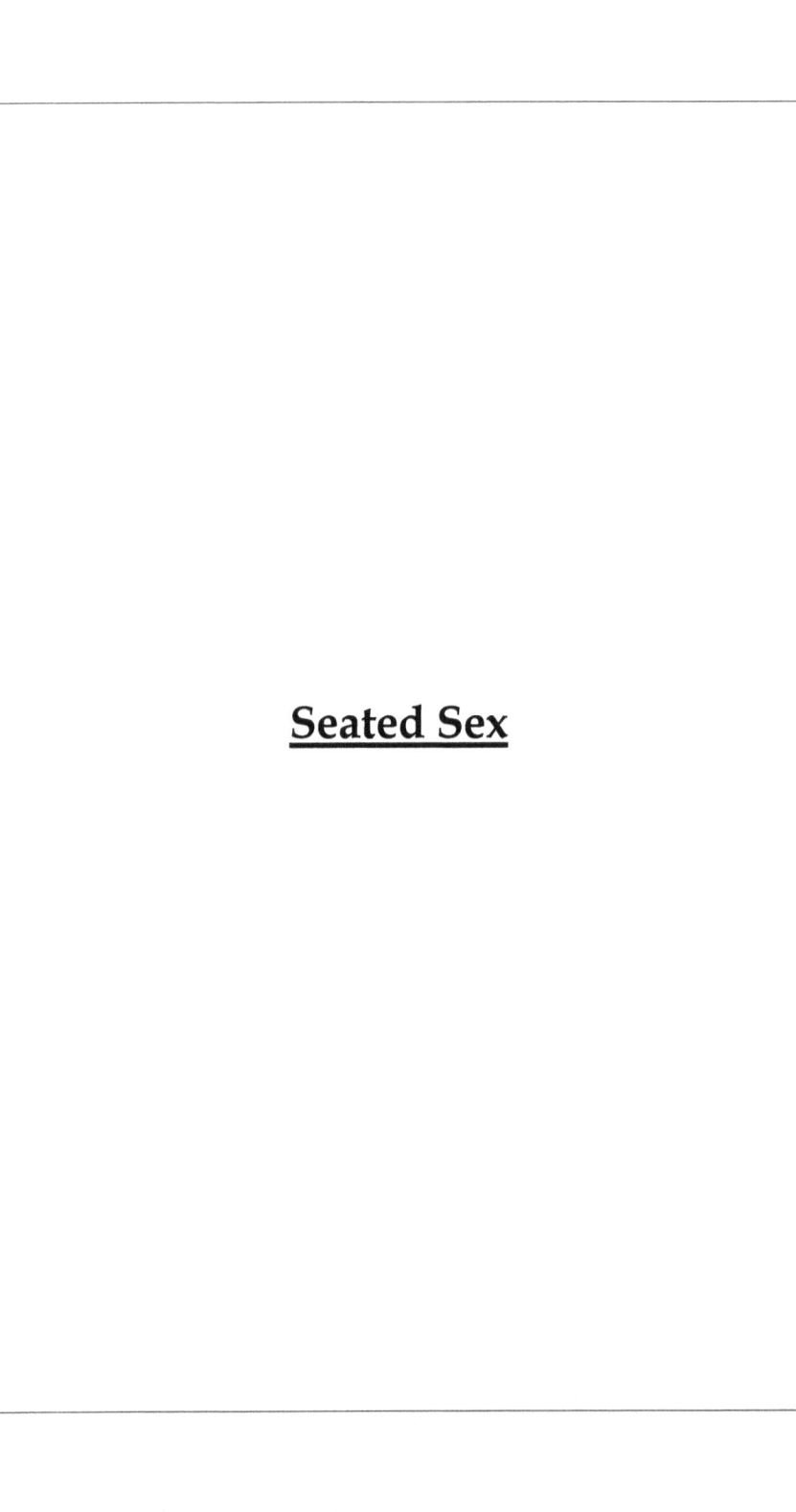

Seated Sex

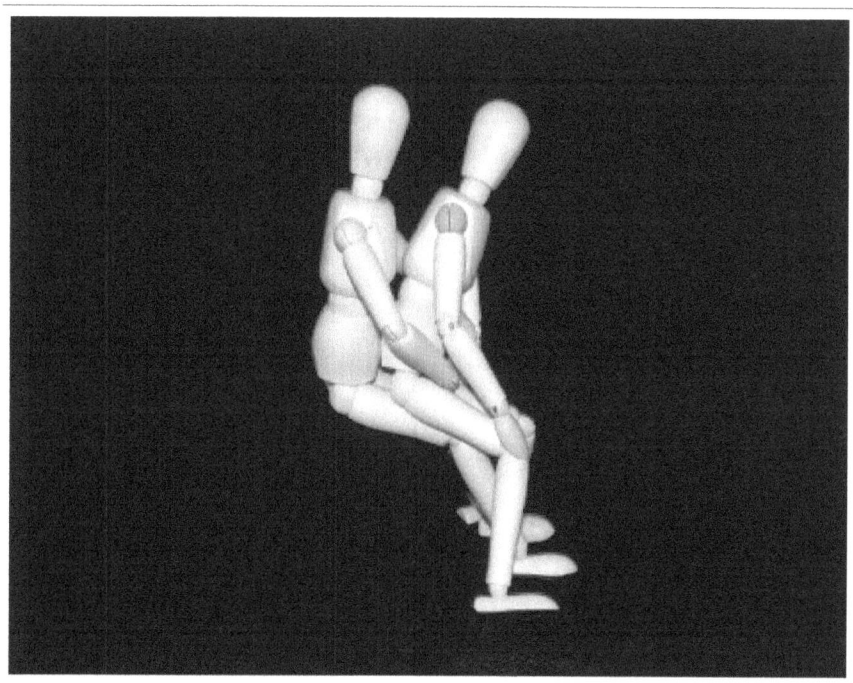

Position Description:

In this position, the man sits on something like a chair, edge of a bed or couch, with an erection. If he is not hard the couple can use the "Big Boss" oral sex position to make sure that he gets fluffed quickly.

Once he is erect, the woman can sit on his lap and slide his cock into her. Once he is inserted, the woman can lift and lower herself onto his cock using her legs, which should be planted firmly on the floor. In this way, she can control the tempo of sex and the depth of penetration.

He on the other hand should hold her and support her while she is fucking him. This can be done either through wrapping his arms around her waist, holding her hips, or by cupping her breasts. If he is cupping her breasts, there is nothing wrong with giving them some attention and stimulation while he is there. They so rarely get enough.

Ease Of Position: Easy

Intimacy Level: Moderate

Wild Spontaneous Level: Moderate

Depth Of Penetration: Deep

Good For Female Orgasm? Yes

Downsides:

The only possible downside to this position is the man just has to lie there and let the woman fuck him. This may be considered a downside to some, but to many couples will be viewed as a plus. An enlightened man will take this opportunity to lavish attention on his partner by running his hands all over her sexy body and kissing her back.

Upsides:

Like with most woman on top positions, this puts the woman firmly in control of the sexual act. She controls everything for a change and can control the speed of sex and the depth of penetration to her comfort. She can make it slow and gentle, or can make it deep, hard and fast and anywhere in between.

Notes On This Position:

This position is a really good one for female orgasm. Since the couple is seated on the edge of a piece of furniture, there is nothing blocking her clitoris, even with him inside her. Even his balls are out of the way thanks to gravity. This means that either partner has wonderful access to stimulate her. This can easily be done with either fingers or a vibrator.

If she is doing the stimulating, it would be recommended that she stop penetration to focus on her orgasm. Instead of moving her body up and down with her legs, she should instead rotate her hips around to move his cock inside of her. This will allow her to focus more on cumming.

If on the other hand she wants his cock jack hammering away, it would be recommended that she focus on moving up and down to increase penetration, while he stimulates her clit. This is a touch harder as it requires coordination and cooperation from the couple. That being said, the two partners working together to make her cum can really bring a couple together and create a sense of unity,

The Piledriver

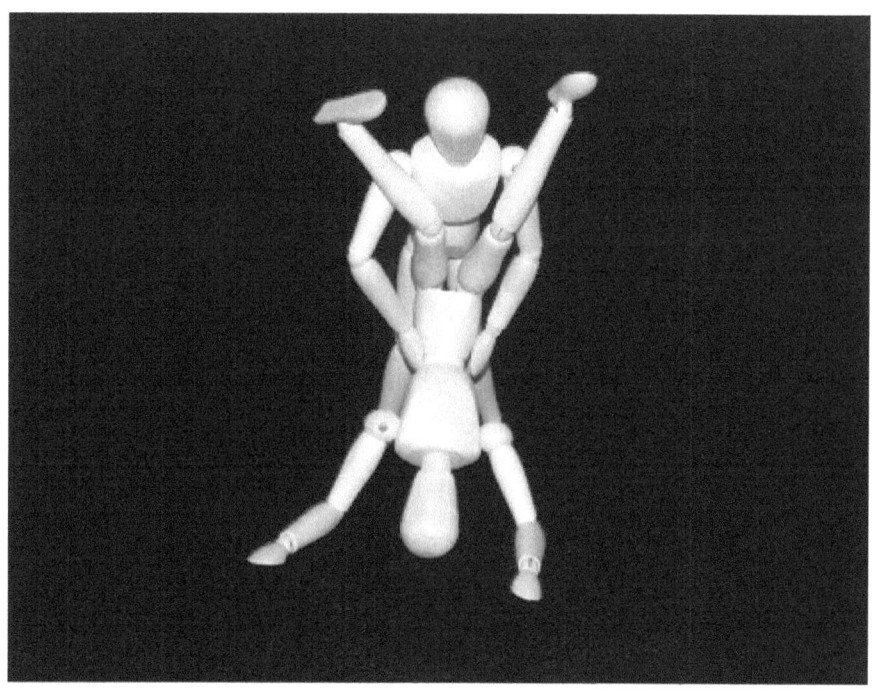

Position Description:

There are two types of piledriver positions. One is intentional and one is accidental.

The accidental piledriver happens when the couple is involved in some kind of missionary position and for one reason or another (usually hard fucking) they slide off the bed or couch. She it winds up on the floor with him still inside her. Usually, because the passion was so high in the first place, the couple just keeps fucking until all the blood rushes to her head. This really is as fun as it sounds and only happens by chance. When it does, the couple should take full advantage of it.

The other type of piledriver is an intentional one.

To assume an intentional piledriver, the woman has a choice. She can either lie on the bed and raise her pelvis above her head with her weight on her head and shoulders or she can lie off the bed with her weight on her head and shoulders and the bed.

The man then assumes a position behind her, lifts her hips to support her and penetrates her. Sex can now begin.

This position can also be entered into from the "Double Handed Buttlift" if the woman raises her pelvis and the man extends his legs at the same time. The couple will then naturally shift into the Piledriver position.

Either way, through out this act, the woman will bear the weight on her head, neck and shoulders and the man should hold onto her hips to help keep her stable.

Ease Of Position: Hard

Intimacy Level: Low

Wild Spontaneous Level: High

Depth Of Penetration: Deep

Good For Female Orgasm? No

Downsides:

Honestly, this position can be pretty uncomfortable for the woman and should be considered more of a novelty position. As a general rule it should only come up during fun sex play and should not be considered a regular part of your lovemaking routine.

Upsides:

Penetration is deep and the man is firmly in control. This makes this position a real turn on for some couples. She is just getting fucked and he is fucking her like some sex starved wild man. It can be fun, but only in small, limited doses.

Notes On This Position:

This position also offer very good access for anal sex. For couple that do like this position, this is something that can be considered.

The T-Bone

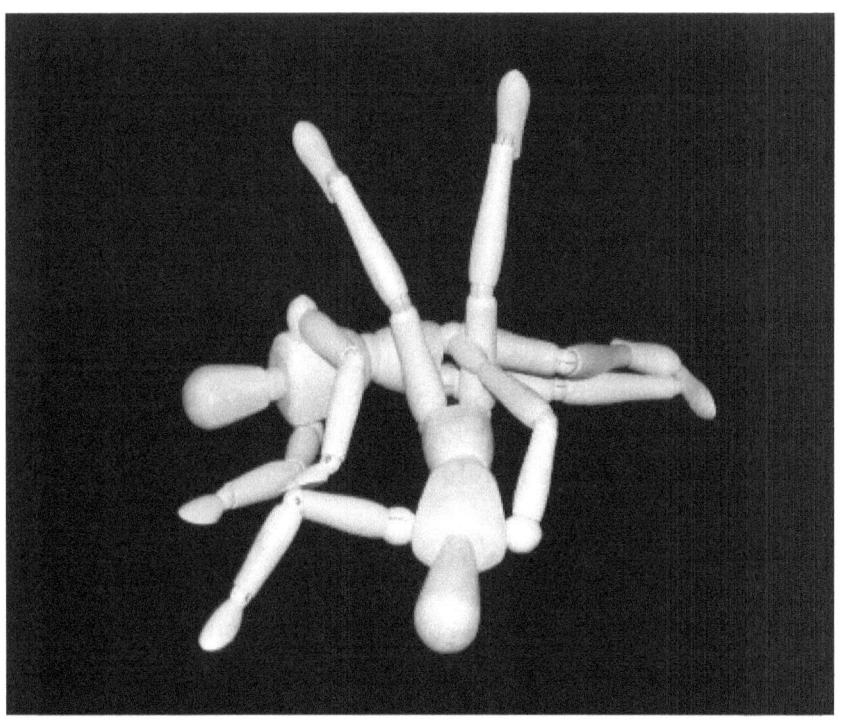

Position Description:

In this position, the man lies on the bed on his side (either one is fine). The woman lies on the bed on her back and raises her legs in the air. His cock should point right at her pussy if the couple is in the right position.

Penetration can now occur as he approaches her and inserts himself. At this point, she can drop her legs over her lover for her comfort. Intercourse can now commence.

Ease Of Position: Moderate

Intimacy Level: High

Wild Spontaneous Level: Moderate

Depth Of Penetration: Shallow

Good For Female Orgasm? Yes

Downsides:

This position does not allow for deep penetration (her butt acts like a cushion and causes shallow penetration) which can slow down or even prevent his orgasm. However, for women whose lovers tend to be quick, this will not be a downside but a huge plus that allows him to take his time.

Upsides:

In this position, the woman is at a great angle to stimulate her clit. The shallow, and thus less vigorous penetration will not interfere and will offer her the chance to possibly cum while her lover is inside her. Many women especially enjoy this position!

Notes On This Position:

The overall tone of this position is slower, gentler, more intimate lovemaking. It is a good way to build and express a bond that exists between a couple. Although he cannot penetrate vigorously or deeply, the head of his cock is inside her, so his pleasure is high and the sensation is wonderful. She on the other hand has a chance to play with herself and look over the whole of her lover's body. This position is a definite visual feast for her.

The physical demands of this position are very low. The lovemaking does not have to be vigorous for either partner to thoroughly enjoy themselves. This is a great position to enjoy when you guys need a break and she maybe needs an orgasm or three.

End To End

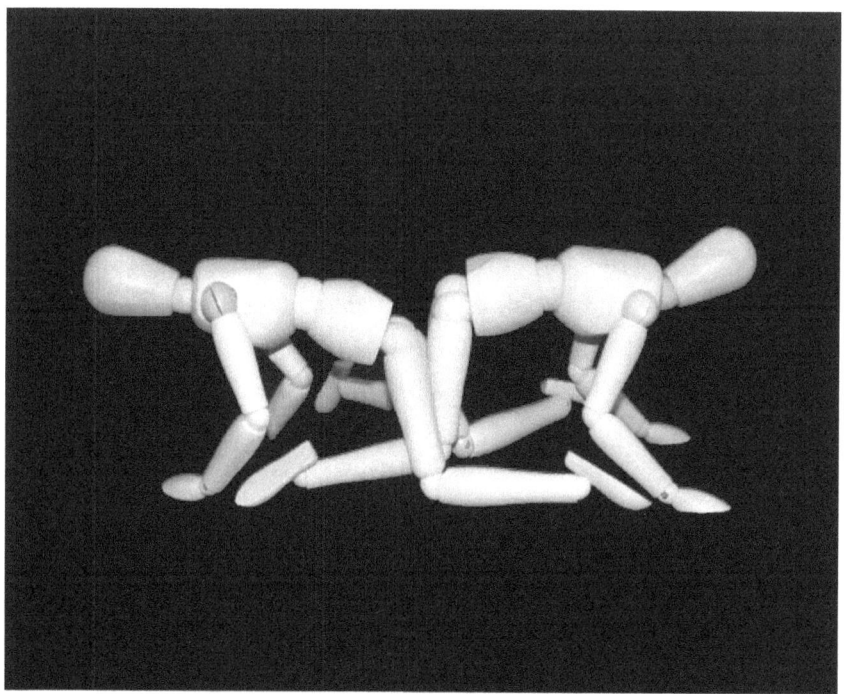

Position Description:

This is one of the positions in this book that is a pure lesbian position. It can only really be performed by two women although some variations are technically possible.

The women begin by each assuming a four point facing away from one another. This means that their pussies are now facing each other.

The two women each insert one end of a double dildo into their vaginas. The dildo is inserted to a comfortable depth.

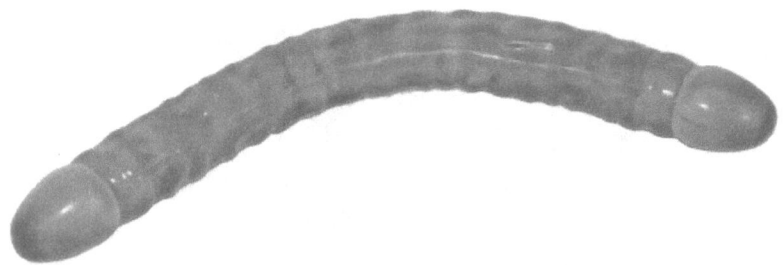

Now, the women can rock back and forth on their knees in unison. This action, creates pressure into their vaginas. With this, the women can "fuck" each other.

They also, can stimulate their clitorises with either their fingers or small vibrators.

Ease Of Position: Easy

Intimacy Level: Moderate

Wild Spontaneous Level: High

Depth Of Penetration: Deep

Good For Female Orgasm? Yes

Downsides:

The biggest downside to this position is that the two women are not facing the same way. This means there is no personal interaction, face to face, eye contact, or kissing. This takes away from the personal connection and can leave either partner feeling disconnected.

Upsides:

This position allows for each woman to be penetrated at the same time. This means that both partners have a chance to orgasm simultaneously. This is rare in lesbian sex, especially with penetration.

Notes On This Position:

Although this position is a little less than practical, however, it can be a lot of fun. Both women are having their vaginas and possibly their clits stimulated simultaneously.

This position also has a lot of show value. It is very appealing to men to watch. If you are acting out a threesome, consider this position as a way to visually entice the man. He will be thinking about it for years to come! You can also modify the position by having either woman performing oral sex for the man. He can even go back and forth until he can't take it anymore and orgasms.

Scissoring

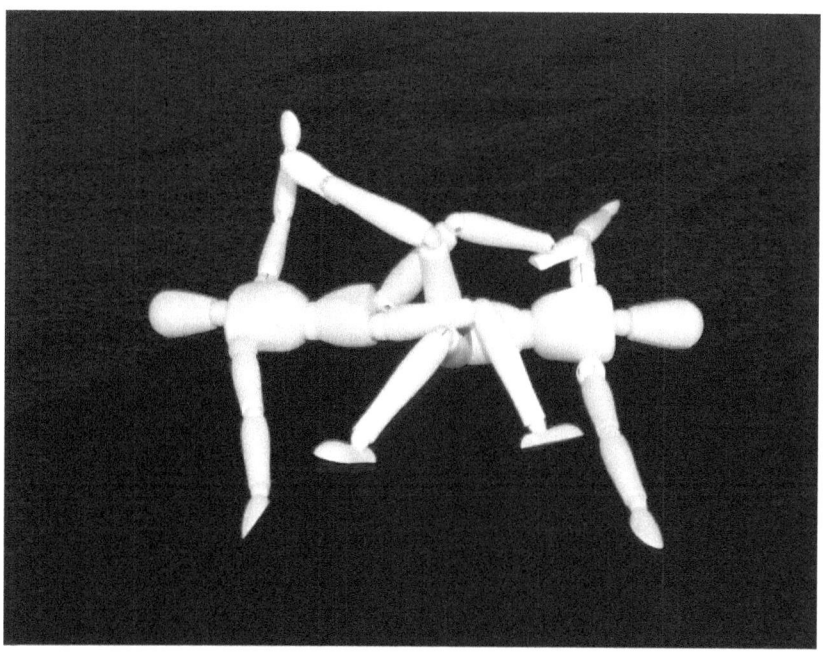

Position Description:
This is also a purely lesbian position. There is nothing here of use to a man.

In this position, one of the women lies on the bed on her back and spreads her legs. Her partner also lies on the bed in the same position, however in an opposite orientation.

At this point, the women's two pussies should be pointing at each other as in the picture above. The women then move close together until their pussies actually touch. From here, the two can rub their pussies together in an intimate act of foreplay or insert a double ended dildo for penetration play.

Ease Of Position: Easy

Intimacy Level: Moderate

Wild Spontaneous Level: Moderate

Depth Of Penetration: N/A (Unless a dildo is used)

Good For Female Orgasm? Possible

Downsides:

With this position, there is no kissing which lowers the bond between the lovers. However, the intimate pussy to pussy contact does create a close bond.

Upsides:

This is a non-oral sex position for lesbians which is very useful. There is even the option for penetration sans a strap on dildo.

Notes On This Position:

This position is often a bit of a joke among men who secretly desire to see two women performing this act. That may be true, but it is also true that this can be a very intimate, very rewarding position for two women. Just because it is so often seen in pornos and comedies as a joke does not mean that there is no place for this very enjoyable position in your sexual routine.